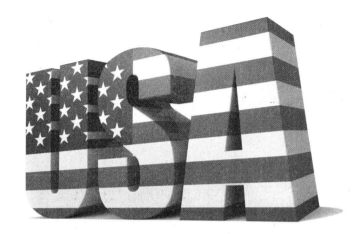

美国急诊

临床必知 200 招

(美)肖锋 / 编著

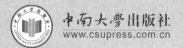
中南大学出版社
www.csupress.com.cn

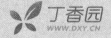
丁香园
WWW.DXY.CN

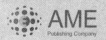
AME
Publishing Company

图书在版编目(CIP)数据

美国急诊临床必知 200 招/肖锋主编 . —长沙:中南大学出版社,
2015. 9

ISBN 978 - 7 - 5487 - 1896 - 3

Ⅰ.美… Ⅱ.肖… Ⅲ.急诊-美国-汉、英 Ⅳ. R4

中国版本图书馆 CIP 数据核字(2015)第 205758 号

美国急诊临床必知 200 招

肖 锋 主编

□责任编辑 郭 征 平静波
□责任印制 易红卫
□出版发行 中南大学出版社
　　　　　　社址:长沙市麓山南路　　　邮编:410083
　　　　　　发行科电话:0731-88876770　　传真:0731-88710482
□印　　装 长沙市宏发印刷有限公司

□开　　本 720×1000 1/16 □印张 32.5 □字数 633 千字
□版　　次 2015 年 9 月第 1 版 □印次 2015 年 9 月第 1 次印刷
□书　　号 ISBN 978 - 7 - 5487 - 1896 - 3
□定　　价 79. 00 元

总序

　　2008 年 4 月，美国急诊医师协会（American College of Emergency Physicians，ACEP）将急诊医学定义为：致力于诊断和治疗不可预见的疾病和外伤。2013 年 ACEP 对急诊医学临床模式（Model of the Clinical Practice of Emergency Medicine）进行了更新，进一步明确了急诊医学实践模式的三维内容，包括急诊医生的业务范畴（Physician Tasks）、患者病情判断（Patient Acuity），及急诊医学临床实践必须掌握的中心内容（Medical Knowledge，Patient Care，Procedural Skills）。国际急诊医学联盟（International Federation of Emergency Medicine，IFEM）认为急诊医学是一门临床学科，其知识和技能用以预防、诊断、治疗所有年龄的患者由于危重或急性疾病以及外伤导致的各类生理和行为紊乱；另外它还包括研究和发展院前及院内急诊医疗体系及其所需的技能。

　　总而言之，急诊医学兼具跨学科和综合性等专业特点。在任何一个国家和地区的医疗体系中，急诊科都是唯一一个处理所有有急性需求患者的前沿阵地。因此，作为一名急诊医生，一定要做到如下几点：知识要博而广；诊断要敏而全；治疗要精而准；操作要快而熟。

　　中国的急诊医学自 20 世纪 80 年代中期作为专科成立以来已经取得了突飞猛进的发展，但在专科建设、科室管理、人员（住院医师）培训、继续教育、临床实践等方面与美国相比还有很大的差距。与医学领域的其他学科相比，急诊医学尽管还很年轻，但其在循证医学方面的发展却日新月异。本系列丛书旨在通过 100 个真实的急诊病例（美国急诊临床病例解析 100 例）、200 个专题讨论（美国急诊临床必知 200 招）、365 个一日一题（美国急诊临床 365 问），向国内同仁及时介绍美国急诊临床标准化实践和基于循证医学的国际急诊医学的最新进展，对临床常见甚至罕见病例以及查房时最常碰到的问题提供科学的解答。同时，希望本系列丛书能够作为医学院临床实习学生、各专业住院医生、基层医生、全科医生、危重病医生、急诊医生，以及任何到急诊科轮转或需要处理急诊病人的其他专科医生必备的参考书。

　　《美国急诊临床荟萃》丛书具备如下特色：

　　1. 循证：及时反应当前美国和基于循证医学的国际急诊医学新理念新实践。

　　2. 短小：一题一答，一问一解，一个病例一个专题。

　　3. 易读：条理清晰，中英对照，是学习医学专业英语不可多得的辅助材料。

4. 实用：能够帮助临床医生解决实际的临床问题。

要了解和学习新的病例、新的必知和新的每日一题，可关注我的微信公共平台（美国急诊临床经验荟萃，或 Dr_XiaoUSA）、我的微博（微博名：Dr_XiaoUS），丁香园急救与危重病专栏（丁香园 ID：Dr_XiaoUS），以及我与《中华急诊医学杂志》和《中国急诊网》合作的专栏：马里兰大学医学院急诊科必知（http://blog.sina.com.cn/s/articlelist_1904076233_14_1.html）。你也可以扫描下面的二维码直接关注。同时欢迎大家通过这几个平台或下面的电子邮箱进行反馈和交流。

感谢 Drs. Brian Browne，Laura Pimentel 和 Fermin Barrueto 对我的支持和帮助。感谢与我同舟共济 25 年的太太（徐燕）和我的两个可爱的儿子（Adam 和 Derek）对我的理解和支持。

Feng Xiao，MD
肖锋，医学博士
美国马里兰医学中心附属 Upper Chesapeake 医院急诊科
北京和睦家医院急诊科
fxiao88@gmail.com
2014 年 8 月 28 日于美国

美
国
急
诊
临
床
必
知
200
招

前　言

　　《美国急诊临床必知 200 招》来自于美国马里兰大学医学中心急诊科权威性的"急诊医学教育必知(Emergency Medicine Educational Pearls)"。马里兰医学中心急诊科拥有 70 多位已经获得急诊医学专科认证的急诊医生,以及多位在国际和国内都享有声誉的急诊医学教育家。同时,本急诊科在急诊住院医师培训方面也具有广泛的知名度。正如急诊科主任 Dr. Brian Browne 教授所说,We train tomorrow's leaders in emergency medicine to positively affect the lives of our patients and to expand our specialty's contributions to patient care(我们培训的,是能够维护患者生命健康和扩展急诊专业对医疗服务贡献的未来急诊医学的领导者)。

　　本书中的这些"必知"均来源于国际上最权威的医学杂志,包括:JAMA(美国医学会杂志)、NEJM(新英格兰医学杂志)、AEM(急诊医学年鉴)、CCM(危重病医学)等。每一条必知的内容,均经过国际著名的马里兰大学医学中心急诊医学专家的编辑和整理。本书的内容精简实用,每一招是反应急诊医学、危重病学以及循证医学最新进展的经典摘要。通过对本书的阅读,你将学习到国际上最新的治疗指南,了解到循证医学的最新进展,并对许多临床问题有新的认识。本书以中英文对照的方式呈现给大家,是学习医学英语不可多得的辅助材料,更是急诊医生在短时间内跟上国际发展步伐必不可少的工具。

　　要了解和学习新的马里兰急诊医学必知,可关注我与《中华急诊医学杂志》和《中国急诊网》合作的专栏:马里兰大学医学院急诊科必知(http://blog. sina. com. cn/s/articlelist_1904076233_14_1. html),我的微博(微博名:Dr_XiaoUS),以及我的微信公共平台(美国急诊临床经验荟萃,或 Dr_XiaoUSA)。你也可以扫描下面的二维码直接关注。同时欢迎大家通过这几个平台或下面的电子邮箱进行反馈和交流。

感谢 Dr. Amal Mattu 教授允许我将这些"必知"的内容介绍给国内急诊医学的同仁以及广大读者。

Feng Xiao，MD
肖锋，医学博士
2014 年 8 月 28 日于美国

目　录

气道管理

心肺复苏

心脏病

危重病

神经疾病

呼吸系统急症

感染性疾病

外科与外伤

国际区域性疾病

药物中毒

急诊操作

灾难医学

其它

气道管理
Airway Management

1. Safer Intubation with a nasal cannula?

1. Pre-oxygenation prior to rapid sequence intubation (RSI) is performed to prevent hypoxemia during endotracheal intubation.

2. An appropriate period of pre-oxygenation will potentially increase the amount of apnea time during intubation, however patients with certain critical illnesses (e. g. , severe pneumonia) may desaturate faster than expected.

3. Apnea time can be increased by maintaining high-flow oxygen by nasal cannula (e. g. , 15 L), during application of the bag-valve mask and during the time of attempted endotracheal tube placement; this concept is known as **apneic oxygenation**.

4. **Apneic oxygenation** is based on the principle that when patients are apneic, alveoli absorb oxygen into the blood stream at a rate of approximately 250 mL/minute, creating a diffusion gradient from the pharynx (containing a high-density of oxygen from the nasal cannula) to a lower concentration of oxygen in the alveoli.

5. Although a patient's oxygenation can be maintained longer using apneic oxygenation, its application does not remove the continuous buildup of CO_2 in the alveoli during apena. Therefore, respiratory acidosis can result after a prolonged period of apneic oxygenation.

Author: **Haney Mallemat**

1. 应用鼻导管辅助气管插管安全吗？

1. 快速顺序插管(RSI)前给氧用于防止气管插管时出现缺氧状态。

2. 适当的插管前给氧能增加插管时的窒息时间，但是一些危重患者(如重型肺炎患者)却会很快进入缺氧状态。

3. 鼻导管高流量(15 L)给氧会增加球囊活门面罩和气管内插管所需的窒息时间，这一概念被称为**窒息性供氧**。

4. **窒息性供氧**的机制是，在窒息时，肺泡氧吸收速度大概为 250 mL/min，从而在高氧浓度的咽喉部与低氧浓度的肺泡之间产生了氧浓度差，引起氧弥散。

5. 虽然窒息性供氧会维持较高的氧含量，但并不能排除由于窒息造成的二氧化碳潴留。因此，长时间的窒息性供氧会产生呼吸性酸中毒。

参考文献：

Weingart, S and Levitan, R. Preoxygenation and prevention of desaturation during emergency airway management. Ann Emerg Med. 2012 Mar; 59(3): 165 – 175. e1

作者：**Haney Mallemat**

气
道
管
理

2. Non-invasive Ventilation (NIV):
What's the Evidence?

1. Emergency Medicine physicians are gaining experience with non-invasive ventilation (i. e. , Bi-level ventilation and continuous positive-pressure ventilation) in managing respiratory distress and failure. Although NIV is commonly used across a variety of pathologies, the best data exists for use with COPD exacerbation and cardiogenic pulmonary edema (CHF, not an acute MI).

2. Although other indications for NIV have been studied, the data is less robust (eg. , smaller study size, weak control groups, etc.). If there are no contraindications, however, many experts still support a trial of NIV in the following populations:

1) Asthma.

2) Severe community acquired pneumonia.

3) Acute lung injury/Acute respiratory distress syndrome.

4) Chest trauma (lung contusion, rib fractures, flail chest, etc).

5) Immunosuppression with acute respiratory failure.

6) Neuromuscular respiratory failure (eg. , Myesthenia Gravis).

7) Cystic Fibrosis.

8) Pneumocystis Jiroveci Pneumonia.

9) "Do not intubate" status.

3. Failure to clinically improve during a NIV trial should prompt invasive mechanical ventilation.

Author: Haney Mallemat

2. 非创伤性(无创)通气(NIV)：
有证据支持吗？

1. 急诊医生在处理呼吸困难或衰竭患者时使用包括双水平气道正压通气(Bi-PAP)和持续气道正压通气(CPAP)的经验越来越丰富。虽然非创伤性通气(NIV)在很多的病理情况下应用，但最有力的证据还是来自于对 COPD 和心源性肺水肿(CHF)恶化时的治疗。

2. 虽然 NIV 在其他方面的应用已有报道，但都由于样本小或对照弱等原因而说服力不足。但如果没有禁忌证，下列情况下专家还是建议考虑使用 NIV：

1)哮喘；

2)危重型院外获得性肺炎；

3)急性肺损伤/急性呼吸窘迫综合征(ARDS)；

4)胸部外伤(肺挫伤，肋骨骨折，连枷胸等)；

5)免疫抑制伴有急性呼吸衰竭；

6)神经肌肉功能紊乱造成的呼吸衰竭(如重症肌无力)；

7)囊肿性纤维化；

8)卡氏肺囊虫肺炎；

9)"放弃抢救"状态。

3. 如使用 NIV 一段时间后临床症状无改善，要及时改用侵入性(插管)机械通气。

参考文献：

Keenan, S. et al. Clinical practice guidelines for the use of noninvasive positive-pressure ventilation and noninvasive continuous positive airway pressure in the acute care setting. CMAJ. 2011 Feb 22；183(3)：E195 – 214. Epub 2011 Feb 14.

作者：**Haney Mallemat**

气道管理

3. Intubation Pearls

When considering an intubation or managing an emergent respiratory concern, keep the "P"s of intubation in mind:

1. Position: No intubating on the floor! Maintain an appropriate distance. Align the airway axes. Sniffing position is utilized for non traumatic adult airways; this involves flexion of the lower c-spine and a bit of extension at the upper cervical levels. Take off cervical collars. Use pillows/blankets to align the external auditory canal (EAC) with the sternal notch to help w/visualization. Cricoid pressure is NOT designed to facilitate passage of the ETT. It MAY help prevent excessive gastric insufflation.

2. Preparation: Two tubes. Two blades. Two intubators. Plan B (ougie) or Plan C (cric). Though your emergency airway plans may differ, think of ALL airways as potentially difficult ones. Respect the epiglottis.

3. Preoxygenation: 100% via NRBM when possible to ensure oxygenation and nitrogen washout. In patinets with at least some reserve, this will help to avoid pulse ox pitfalls. True RSI does NOT involve positive pressure ventilation.

4. Premedication: Know your sedatives in advance. Etomidate? Ketamine? Diprivan? Whatever your agent of choice, know indications and drug dosages. Emergent RSI is a less than ideal time to access Epocrates.

5. Paralysis: This is pretty much the point of no return. Administration of paralytics commits you to securing a patient's airway. Both rocuronium and succynylcholine can be dosed at 1 mg/kg IV.

6. Pass the tube

7. Position confirmation: Direct visualization of the tube through the glottic opening coupled with end tidal CO_2 is ideal.

Author: Benjamin Lawner

美
国
急
诊
临
床
必
知
200
招

6

3.气管插管的要点

在考虑要插管或抢救急性呼吸困难患者时，要记住几个与插管有关的"P"：

1.位置(Position)：千万不要在地板上插管！保持适当的距离。对齐呼吸道轴线。非创伤成年患者可使用"嗅物位"，使患者下部颈椎前屈而上部颈椎后仰，解开患者颈托，用枕头和毯子将其外耳道和胸骨切迹对齐以帮助医生直视(声门)。环状软骨加压并不是用来帮助放置气管导管的，它可能能防止大量胃内容物反流导致窒息。

2.准备(Preparation)：两个导管，两个喉镜，两个操作人。要准备好计划 B (Bougie，弹性引导管芯)和计划 C(Cric，气管切开)。虽然急诊呼吸道处理的方案不同，但一定要把所有的呼吸道都作为困难呼吸道处理。对会厌要引起重视。

3.前期给氧(Preoxygenation)：在可能情况下，为保证供氧和排出氮气，要通过非呼吸器面罩输 100% 的氧。真正的快速顺序插管并不需要正压通气。

4.操作前给药(Premedication)：要提前掌握你的镇静药，依托咪酯？氯胺酮？或异丙酚？无论你的选择是什么，要了解它们的适应证和剂量。急诊情况下，你不可能有时间再查 Epocrates(参考文献)。

5.肌肉松弛(Paralysis)：这时你不可能再回头了。给了肌松药你就必须要保护患者的呼吸道。罗库溴铵和琥珀酰胆碱都可以按1mg/kg 静注。

6.放入导管(Pass the tube)

7.证实位置(Position confirmation)：最好要在直视声门并监测呼吸末期 CO_2 的情况下进行插管。

作者：Benjamin Lawner

气
道
管
理

4. Paralytic Agents for RSI

1. Emergency Physicians regularly use neuromuscular blocking agents for rapid sequence intubation. It is not uncommon to wonder why a specific patient seems to respond with inadequate paralysis or an extended duration of neuromuscular blockade. Some pearls regarding the use of nondepolarizing agents:

1) Hypercalcemia decreases duration of blockade.

2) Hypermagnesemia prolongs the duration of action.

3) Hypothermia can prolong the duration of action.

4) Hypokalemia may augment the blockade.

5) Acidosis enhances the blockade effect.

2. Aminoglycosides are known to prolong the duration of action. Patients chronically on phenytoin/carbamazepine exhibit resistance to rocuronium.

3. Severe hepatic dysfunction prolongs rocuronium's effect. However, renal failure does not affect the duration of single doses.

Author: Feng Xiao

美
国
急
诊
临
床
必
知
200
招

4. 快速顺序插管(RSI)时肌松剂的使用

1. 急诊医师经常在做 RSI 时使用神经肌肉阻断药。值得思考的是为什么患者不是反应不足就是出现神经肌肉阻滞的持续时间延长。下面是几个在使用非去极化肌松剂时的要点：

1) 高钙血症缩短阻滞时间。

2) 高镁血症将延长有效时间。

3) 低温可以延长有效时间。

4) 低钾血症可增强阻滞效果。

5) 酸中毒加强阻滞的效果。

2. **氨基苷类抗生素**延长有效时间是众所周知的。长期服用苯妥英钠/卡马西平的患者会出现对罗库溴铵的耐药。

3. 严重肝功能障碍可延长罗库溴铵的作用。然而，肾功能衰竭并不影响单剂量的持续时间。

参考文献：

(1) Greenberg SB, et al. Crit Care Med 2013；41：1332 – 1344.

(2) Warr J, et al. Ann Pharmacother 2011；45：1116 – 1126.

作者：肖锋(Feng Xiao)

气道管理

9

5. Intubating an Obese Patient

1. The supine position during rapid sequence intubation may result in posterior lung atelectasis thereby reducing lung volumes, oxygenation reserve, and ultimately apnea time.

2. Several studies have shown that elevating the head of the bed by at least 20 degrees or placing a patient in reverse Trendelenberg position (for patients with contra-indications to elevating the head of the bed) during RSI may significantly increase apnea time.

3. Elevating the head of the bed may be especially helpful for patients with BMIs >35.

Author: Haney Mallemat

5. 肥胖患者气管插管

1.在快速顺序插管时，平卧位所造成的肺后叶的肺不张可导致肺容量和肺氧储备量降低，使窒息时间缩短。

2.有一些临床研究显示：将床头抬高至少20°或将患者处于反Trendelenburg位（如果不允许将患者头部抬高），可以在快速顺序插管时明显延长窒息时间。

3.抬高床头对体质指数（BMI）大于35的患者尤其有效。

参考文献：

Weingart，S and Levitan，R. Preoxygenation and prevention of desaturation during emergency airway management. Ann Emerg Med. 2012 Mar；59（3）：165－175. el.

作者：**Haney Mallemat**

气道管理

6. Postintubation Hypotension

1. It is clear that preintubation hypotension is associated with increased mortality in critically ill patients who require mechanical ventilation.

2. Unfortunatley, the literature is less clear on the frequency and impact of hypotension that develops after intubation.

3. Two recent publications in the Journal of Intensive Care provide valuable information on postintubation hypotension. Some highlights of the studies include:

1) Retrospective cohorts of over 300 patients who developed postintubation hypotension, defined as a SBP $<$90 mm Hg within 60 min of intubation.

2) Postintubation hypotension occurred in almost 25% of patients.

3) Median time to hypotension was 11 minutes.

4) Patients with postintubation hypotension had a higher inhospital mortality (33% vs. 23%).

5) A preintubation Shock Index $>$0. 8 was the strongest predictor of cardiovascular collapse after intubation.

4. Take Home Point: Postintubation hypotension occurs frequently and may be associated with worse outcomes.

Author: Michael Winters

美
国
急
诊
临
床
必
知
200
招

6. 插管后的低血压

1.已经非常清楚的是，对于需要气管插管的危重患者，插管前低血压与死亡率增加有关。

2.遗憾的是，对于插管后低血压的发生频率和后果并没有明确的报道。

3.最新发表在美国《危重病学杂志》上的两篇文章，为插管后的低血压提供了有价值的信息。其中要点列举如下：

1)这些回顾性研究包括插管后60分钟内发生低血压(收缩压低于90 mmHg)的300余例患者。

2)接近25%的患者出现插管后低血压。

3)低血压的出现时间平均在11分钟。

4)出现插管后低血压的患者住院期间死亡率较高(33%与23%)。

5)插管前休克指数大于0.8是预测发生插管后循环衰竭的最有效指标。

4.注意

气管插管后低血压非常常见，并与不良预后有关。

参考文献：

Heffner AC, Swords D, Kline JA, et al. The frequency and significance of postintubation hypotension during emergency airway management. J Crit Care 2012；27：417e9 – 417e13.

Heffner AC, Swords D, Nussbaum ML, et al. Predictors of the complication of postintubation hypotension during emergency airway management. J Crit Care 2012；27：587 – 593.

作者：**Michael Winters**

7. What is the Lowest Tidal Volume?

1. A low-tidal volume (or protective) strategy of mechanical ventilation (i. e. , tidal volume of 6 – 8cc/kg of ideal body weight) has previously been demonstrated to be beneficial in patients with acute respiratory distress syndrome (ARDS).

2. A meta-analysis was recently performed to determine whether this strategy of mechanical ventilation is also beneficial for patients without lung injury prior to initiation of mechanical ventilation.

3. Dr. Neto, et al. performed a meta-analysis of 20 studies (total of 2, 822 mechanically ventilated patients) comparing a conventional ventilation strategy (average tidal volume was 10. 6 cc/kg) to a protective ventilation strategy (average tidal volume was 6. 4 cc/kg) of mechanical ventilation.

The authors concluded that patients ventilated with a protective lung-strategy had reductions in:

1) Mortality.

2) Lung injury and ARDS.

3) Atelectasis.

4) Pulmonary infections.

5) Length of hospital stay.

4. **Bottom-line**: This meta-analysis supports the notion that a strategy of low-tidal volume ventilation may have benefits for patients without ARDS, however prospective studies are needed.

Author: Haney Mallemat

7.最低潮气量会是多少?

1. 机械通气时采用低潮气量(保护性)方案(即潮气量在每公斤标准体重 6~8 毫升)在过去治疗急性呼吸窘迫综合征已经被证实是有效的。

2. 最近,有人作了一项 Meta 分析,以确定此机械通气方案是否也可以用于未使用呼吸机前无肺损伤的患者。

3. Neto 等医生对 20 篇文献(一共有 2 822 个机械通气的患者)进行了分析报告,对传统通气方案(平均潮气量为 10.6 mL/kg)与保护性机械通气方案(平均潮气量为 6.4 mL/kg)进行了比较。

作者指出,保护性低潮气量方案可减少以下并发症和相关指标:

1)死亡率。

2)肺损伤和 ARDS。

3)肺不张。

4)肺部感染。

5)住院时间。

4. **要点**

该 Meta 分析结果进一步提示,低潮气量通气可应用于没有 ARDS 的患者。但还需要前瞻性的临床试验进一步证实。

参考文献:

Neto, S. et al. Association between use of lung-protective ventilation with lower tidal volumes and clinical outcomes among patients without acute respiratory distress syndrome. JAMA, Oct. 24/31; 308; 16.

作者: **Haney Mallemat**

气道管理

8. Don't Fall Asleep on Auto-PEEP

1. Mechanically ventilated patients can develop a condition in which air becomes trapped within the alveoli at end-expiration; this is called auto-PEEP.

2. Auto-peep has several adverse effects:

1) Barotrauma from positive pressure trapped within the alveoli.

2) Increased work of breathing.

3) Worsening pulmonary gas exchange.

4) Hemodynamic compromise secondary to increased intra-thoraic pressure.

3. Auto-PEEP classically occurs in intubated patients with asthma or emphysema, but it may also occur in the absence of such disease. The risk of auto-PEEP is increased in patients with:

1) Short expiration times (i. e. , inadequate time for the evacuation of alveolar air at end-expiration).

2) Bronchoconstriction.

3) Plugging of the bronchi (e. g. , mucus or foreign body) creating a one-way valve and air-trapping.

4. Auto-PEEP may be treated by:

1) Reducing tidal volume.

2) Reducing the respiratory rate.

3) Decreasing inspiratory time.

4) Increasing PEEP.

5) Patients may need to be heavily sedated to accomplish the above ventilator maneuvers.

Author: Haney Mallemat

8.不要小看内源性呼气末正压(PEEP)

1.机械通气的患者会出现肺泡内气体在呼气末的潴留,这一现象称为内源性呼气末正压。

2.内源性呼气末正压有几个不良反应:

1)由肺泡内产生的正压力造成的压力损伤。

2)增加呼吸负荷。

3)增加肺气体交换阻力。

4)由胸内压的增加所造成的血流动力学紊乱。

3.内源性呼气末正压通常在机械通气的哮喘或肺气肿患者中发生,但也可在没有这些疾病时出现。内源性呼气末正压产生的危险因素有:

1)呼气时间短,没有足够的时间将呼吸末期肺泡内气体清除。

2)支气管痉挛。

3)支气管栓子形成(如黏液或异物),形成止回阀结构和气体滞留。

4.内源性呼气末正压的治疗办法:

1)降低潮气量。

2)减少呼吸频率。

3)缩短吸气时间。

4)增加 PEEP。

5)为达到如上的目标,可能需要对患者进行深度镇静。

作者:Haney Mallemat

气道管理

9. Finding the AutoPEEP

There are 3 ways you can look for evidence of Auto-PEEP on the ventilator:

1. Do an end-expiratory hold: If the measured PEEP is more than the PEEP set on the vent after a 2 – 3 second hold, the difference is your Auto-PEEP.

2. Look at the expiratory flow waveform: If the waveform does not return to baseline (still expiring when inspiratory ventilation occurs), there's Auto-PEEP!

3. Compare the inspiratory vs. expiratory volumes. If the inspiratory volumes are much higher than the expiratory volumes, consider Auto-PEEP.

Author: John Greenwood

9. 如何判断内源性 PEEP

有 3 种方法可以判断使用呼吸机时是否存在内源性 PEEP：

1. 做一个呼气末暂停。如果在暂停 2 ~ 3 s 后测得的呼气末正压超过了呼吸机设定的 PEEP，其差值就是内源性 PEEP。

2. 检查呼气期流速波形。如果波形不回到基线(呼吸机通气时，患者还处于呼气状态)，说明有内源性 PEEP!

3. 比较呼气和吸气容量。如果吸气量明显高于呼气量，要考虑内源性 PEEP。

参考文献：

Blanch L, Bernabé F, Lucangelo U. Measurement of air trapping, intrinsic positive end-expiratory pressure, and dynamic hyperinflation in mechanically ventilated patients[J]. Respir Care. 2005; 50 (1): 110 – 123.

作者：John Greenwood

气道管理

10. Detecting and managing ventilator emergencies

1. There are several reasons why a mechanically ventilated patient may decompensate post-intubation. Immediate action is often needed to reverse the problem, but it can be difficult to remember where to start as the vent alarm is sounding and the patient is decompensating.

2. Consider using the mnemonic "D. O. P. E. S. like D. O. T. T. S. " to assist you in first diagnosing the problem (D. O. P. E. S.) and then fixing the problem (D. O. T. T. S.).

1) Step 1: Could this decompensation be secondary to D. O. P. E. S. ?

(1) Displaced ET tube / ET tube cuff not inflated or has a leak.

(2) Obstruction of ET tube.

(3) Pneumothorax.

(4) Equipment malfunction (disconnection of the ventilator, incorrect vent settings, etc.).

(5) Stacking (breath stacking/Auto-PEEP).

2) Step 2: Fix the problem with D. O. T. T. S.

(1) Disconnect-Disconnect patient from the ventilator.

(2) Oxygen-Oxygenate patient with a BVM and feel for resistance as you bag.

(3) Tube position/function-Did the ET tube migrate? Is it kinked or is there a mucus plug?

(4) Tweak the vent-Are the settings correct for this patient?

(5) Sonogram (ultrasound)-Sonogram to look for pneumothorax, mainstem intubation, etc.

Author: Haney Mallemat

10. 呼吸机患者紧急情况的诊断和处理

1. 机械通气患者在插管后病情加重可能有好几种原因,通常需要做紧急处理。但在呼吸机发出警报和患者情况恶化的状态下,迅速弄清楚如何处理是有一定困难的。

2. 可以考虑用助记口诀"D.O.P.E.S like D.O.T.T.S"帮助你首先发现问题(D.O.P.E.S),然后解决问题(D.O.T.T.S)。

1)第一步:病情加重是否由 D.O.P.E.S 引起?

(1)气管导管位置错误/导管气囊没有充气或漏气。

(2)气管导管阻塞。

(3)气胸。

(4)仪器故障(连接不良,呼吸机设置不正确等)。

(5)叠加效应(呼吸叠加/内源性 PEEP)。

2)第二步:用 D.O.T.T.S 解决问题

(1)断开。解除患者与呼吸机的连接。

(2)给氧。用呼吸囊活瓣面罩给氧,捏球囊时要感觉气道阻力。

(3)检查导管的位置和功能。导管有无错位? 是否有扭结或黏液栓?

(4)调节呼吸机。呼吸机设定对这个患者是否正确?

(5)超声。超声检查以发现气胸、插管过深等。

作者:**Haney Mallemat**

11. Extubating in the ED

1. With the increasing LOS for many of our intubated critically ill ED patients, it is possible that select patients may be ready for extubation while still in the ED.

2. Patients who remain intubated unnecessarily are at increased risk for pneumonia, increased hospital LOS, and increased mortality.

3. To be considered for extubation, patients should meet the following criteria:

1) The condition that resulted in intubation is improved or resolved.

2) Hemodynamically stable (off pressors).

3) $PaO_2/FiO_2 > 200$ with PEEP < 5 cm H_2O.

4. If these criteria are met, perform a spontaenous breathing trial (SBT).

1) Discontinue sedation.

2) Adjust the ventilator to minimal settings: pressure support or CPAP (5 cm H_2O) or use a T-piece.

3) Perform the trial for at least 30 minutes.

5. If the patient develops a RR > 35 bpm, SpO_2 < 90%, HR > 140 bpm, SBP > 180 mm Hg or < 90 mm Hg, or increased anxiety, the SBT ends and the patient should remain intubated.

6. Before removing the endotracheal tube, be sure to assess mentation, the quantity of secretions, and strength of cough.

Author: Michael Winters

美
国
急
诊
临
床
必
知
200
招

11. 在急诊科的气管拔管

1. 很多在急诊科插管的危重患者由于滞留时间长，其中有些人在急诊科就可以拔管。

2. 继续保留不必要的气管插管将增加患者肺炎发病率、住院时间和死亡率。

3. 拔管应满足下列条件：

1）导致插管的病因有改善或治愈。

2）血流动力学稳定（脱离升压药）。

3）血氧浓度/供氧浓度分数比大于 200，PEEP 小于 5 cm H_2O。

4. 如满足这些条件，要进行自主呼吸试验（SBT）。

1）停用镇静药。

2）将呼吸机条件降到最低：压力支持或 CPAP 小于 5 cm H_2O 或用 T 管

3）SBT 试验至少要进行 30 分钟。

5. 如患者的呼吸超过 35 次/min，氧饱和度低于 90%，心率快于 140 次/min，收缩压高于 180 mmHg 或低于 90 mmHg，或焦虑加重，应停止 SBT，继续保持插管。

6. 在拔管前，一定要检查患者的神志、分泌物的量和咳嗽的力度。

参考文献：

McConville JF, Kress JP. Weaning patients from the ventilator. NEJM 2012；367：2233 – 9.

作者：**Michael Winters**

气
道
管
理

12. Does a cuff-leak mean anything?

1. Intubated patients may occasionally meet certain criteria for extubation while in the Emergency Department. Extubation is not without its risk, however, as up to 30% of patients have respiratory distress secondary to laryngeal and upper airway edema, with some patients requiring re-intubation.

2. Prior to extubation, Intensivists use a brief "cuff-leak" test (deflation of the endotracheal balloon to assess the presence or absence of an air-leak around the tube) to indirectly screen for the presence of upper airway edema and ultimately the risk of re-intubation. The cuff-leak test is performed by deflating the endotracheal balloon followed by one or more of the following maneuvers:

1) Using the ventilator to measure the difference between inspired and expired tidal volumes; if there is a difference in the measured volumes, then air is "leaking" around the endotracheal tube, implying minimal airway edema.

2) Auscultation for an air "leak" around the tube during mechanical ventilation; auscultation of a leak implies that air is passing around the tube and minimal airway edema is present.

3) Disconnecting the patient from the ventilator and occluding the endotracheal tube during spontaneous breathing; auscultation of a leak implies that there is air passing around the tube and minimal airway edema is present.

3. Ochoa et al. performed a systematic review to determine the accuracy of the "cuff-leak" test to predict upper airway edema prior to extubation. The authors concluded that a positive cuff-leak test (i. e. , absence of an air-leak) indicates an elevated risk of upper airway obstruction and re-intubation. A negative cuff-leak test (i. e. , presence of an air-leak), however, does not reliably exclude the presence of upper airway edema or the need for subsequent re-intubation.

4. Bottom line: No test prior to extubation reliably predicts the absence of upper airway edema. Patients extubated in the Emergency Department require close observation with airway equipment located nearby.

Author: Haney Mallemat

12. 气囊放气在拔管中有什么意义？

1. 在急诊科插管的患者有时会达到拔管的标准。拔管并不是没有危险的，约30%的患者会因为拔管后喉头和上呼吸道水肿出现呼吸困难，有的患者可能需要再次插管。

2. 医生在拔管前通常要进行一个短暂的"气囊放气"试验（通过气管导管气囊放气以确定是否导管气囊周围有漏气的现象），间接发现上呼吸道水肿的存在，进而确定再插管的危险性。气囊放气试验在放掉气管导管气囊后，应用如下的一个或几个方法判断：

1）用呼吸机来测量吸气和呼气时的潮气量差别，如有差别，则证实气管导管周围有漏气，提示没有明显的气道水肿。

2）用听诊的方式检查机械通气时导管周围，如有漏气，则证实气管导管周围有气体通过，提示没有明显的气道水肿。

3）断开呼吸机，在患者自主呼吸时堵住气管导管，如听到漏气，则证实气管导管周围有气体通过，提示没有明显的气道水肿。

3. Ochoa 等人发表了一篇文献综述，以确定用"气囊放气"试验预测拔管前气道水肿的存在的准确性。他们的结论是，阳性结果（没有漏气）意味着上呼吸道梗阻和再插管的可能性很高，而阴性结果并不能够排除上呼吸道水肿或再插管的可能性。

4. 结论：在拔管前，没有任何一个试验可以可靠地预测不存在上呼吸道水肿。因此，在急诊科拔管后，要对患者进行严密观察，并将呼吸机放在附近。

参考文献：

Ochoa, ME et al. Cuff-leak test for the diagnosis of upper airway obstruction in adults: A systematic review and meta-analysis. Intensive Care Med (2009) 35: 1171 – 1179.

作者：**Haney Mallemat**

气道管理

13. Pediatric intubation

1. When intubating an infant, a few key points need to be kept in mind:

1) Remember that the narrowest point is the cricoid, so even if the ETT passes the cords it might still not pass through the cricoid itself.

2) Remember premedication with atropine is recommended in all children less than 1 year old and in those less than 5 years old when using succinylcholine. It is used to prevent reflex bradycardia and high ICP and to decrease secretions. The dose is 0. 02 mg/kg IV, with a minimum of 0. 1 mg and a max of 0. 5 mg. Give it 2 full minutes before the start of intubation.

3) Remember that succinylcholine is contraindicated in neuromuscular disease (including an undiagnosed myopathy). A slightly higher dose (2 mg/kg) may need to be used in infants (compared to 1 – 1. 5 mg/kg in adults and older children).

4) Pressure control mode is preferred over volume control (VC) setting in peds, because VC tends to overestimate how much volume it's delivering, therefore delivering inadequate ventilation.

2. Remember your alternatives: High Flow Nasal cannula (HFNC) can be used in infants with respiratory distress to avoid intubation. One study showed that is decreased intubation rates by 68% in respiratory distress due to bronchiolitis.

Author: Mimi Lu

13. 小儿气管插管

1. 当给一个婴儿插管时, 需要注意如下几项:

1) 气管最狭窄的部位是环状软骨, 即使气管导管通过了声门, 也不能保证通过环状软骨。

2) 对 1 岁以内或 5 岁以内但要用琥珀胆碱的儿童插管前要给阿托品。主要是为了防止反射性心动过缓, 增加颅压和减少分泌物。平均剂量是 0.02 mg/kg 静脉注射, 最少 0.1 mg, 最大量 0.5 mg。插管前 2 分钟用。

3) 琥珀胆碱在有神经肌肉疾病(包括诊断不明确的肌病)时是禁用的。婴儿的剂量(2 mg/kg)要比大一点的孩子和成人(1～1.5 mg/kg)高一点。

4) 由于容量控制型呼吸模式会高估输出容量, 从而导致通气不足, 因此首先要考虑用压力控制型呼吸机模式。

2. 要记住其他的选择: 为避免气管插管, 对呼吸困难的婴儿可使用高流量鼻导管给氧。有研究显示: 此方法在治疗由细支气管炎导致的呼吸困难时可以减少 68% 的气管插管率。

参考文献:

1. Santillanes G, Gausche-Hill M. Pediatric Airway Management. Emerg Med Clin N Am 26 (2008) 961 – 975

2. Bledsoe G H, Schexnayder S M. Pediatric Rapid Sequence Intubation A Review. Ped Emerg Care 20 (2004) 339 – 344

作者: **Mimi Lu**

气道管理

心肺复苏
Cardiopulmonary Resuscitation

14. Chest compression only CPR

1. Early CPR performed by laypersons can double the chances of survival in out-of-hospital cardiac arrest (OHCA).

2. A retrospective cohort that combined 2 RCT compared the survival effects of dispatcher CPR instruction consisting of chest compression alone or chest compression with rescue breathing.

3. There was a lower risk of death after adjustment for confounders (adjusted hazard ratio 0.91, 95% confidence interval 0.83 − 0.99, p = 0.02).

4. Findings strongly support a long-term mortality benefit of dispatcher CPR instruction strategy consisting of chest compression alone rather than chest compression plus rescue breathing.

Author: SemharTewelde

14. 只有心脏按压的心肺复苏

1. 在入院前心脏骤停中，早期非医护人员进行的心肺复苏能使患者生存率翻一番。

2. 一篇回顾性的临床报告对两个随机临床实验进行了总结，比较了在调度员指导下的单独心脏按压与心脏按压和通气同时进行的效果。

3. 在对影响因素进行调整后，（单独心脏按压组）死亡率明显降低（调整后的危险比为 0.91, 95% 置信区间为 0.83 ~ 0.99, $P = 0.02$）。

4. 结果证实，由调度员指导下的单独心脏按压方案，而不是心脏按压和通气同步进行方案，有益于降低长期死亡率。

参考文献：

Dumas F, Rea T, et al. Chest compression alone cardiopulmonary resuscitation is associated with better long-term survival compared with standard cardiopulmonary resuscitation. Circulation. 2013 Jan 29；127(4)：435 – 441.

作者：SemharTewelde

心肺复苏

15. Improve your Resuscitation!
Tools for the Resus Room

1. Want to improve your chances of success in the resus room? Download a metronome app on your smartphone and set it to a rate of 100 – 120 beats per minute. There are a number of cheap (usually free) metronome applications for both iOS and Android devices.

2. A recent review looked at the evidence behind CPR feedback devices and found:

1) Compared to baseline, chest compression rates and end-tidal CO_2 improved after activation of the metronomes.

2) There was a significant improvement in the hands-off time per minute during CPR.

3) The proportion of intubation attempts taking under 20 seconds improved.

4) There were increased survival rates when implemented in the pre-hospital setting.

3. So go over to the App store and download a free metronome. Your resus team will be able to stay on track with their compressions and even better-they won't have to hear you sing!

Author: John Greenwood

15. 提高你的心肺复苏率! 抢救室必备的工具

1. 想要提高抢救室的复苏成功率吗? 在智能手机应用程序中下载一个节拍器, 将速度设置为 100 ~ 120 次/min。有许多便宜(甚至是免费的)并与 iOS 和 Android 设备兼容的节拍器。

2. 一篇文献回顾对在 CPR 时应用反馈装置的证据进行了分析, 发现:

1) 与基线相比, 在应用节拍器后胸外按压频率和呼气末 CO_2 都有改善。

2) 在心肺复苏过程中, 每分钟手离开时间有显著的改善。

3) 20 秒内插管成功比例提高。

4) 在院前就使用可增加存活率。

3. 所以, 到 App 店下载一个免费的节拍器, 你的复苏团队将能够掌握他们的按压频率——他们不需要再听你唱歌了!

参考文献:

Yeung J, Meeks R, Edelson D, Gao F, Soar J, Perkins GD. The use of CPR feedback/prompt devices during training and CPR performance: A systematic review[J]. Resuscitation. 2009 Jul; 80 (7): 743 – 751.

作者: **John Greenwood**

心肺复苏

16. Mechanical vs. Manual Chest Compressions

1. A recent meta-analysis of 12 studies (6, 538 patients with 1, 824 ROSC) assessed the quality of cardiopulmonary resuscitation (CPR) using either manual vs. mechanical (load-distributing or piston-driven) compressions in out-of-hospital cardiac arrest.

2. Compared w/manual CPR, load-distributing band CPR had significantly greater odds of ROSC (odds ratio, 1. 62 and $p < 0.001$).

3. The treatment effect for piston-driven CPR was similar to manual CPR.

4. The difference in percentages of ROSC rates from CPR was 8. 3% for load-distributing band CPR and 5. 2% for piston-driven CPR.

5. Compared with manual CPR, combining both mechanical CPR devices produced a significant treatment effect in favor of higher odds of ROSC with mechanical CPR devices (odds ratio, 1. 53 and $p < 0.001$).

Author: Semhar Tewelde

16. 机械与人工胸外按压

1. 最近的一项 Meta 分析报告对 12 项用人工和机械(负荷均匀按压带或驱动活塞)按压心肺复苏(CPR)的院外心脏骤停研究(6 538 例患者,其中 1 824 自主循环恢复(ROSC))进行了质量评估。

2. 与手动 CPR 相比,负荷均匀按压带可明显提高 ROSC(比值比为 1.62,$P < 0.001$)。

3. 活塞驱动 CPR 的治疗效果与人工 CPR 类似。

4. 负荷均匀按压带 CPR 心肺复苏 ROSC 率的差异百分比为 8.3%,而活塞驱动 CPR 为 5.2%。

5. 与人工 CPR 相比,这两个机械心肺复苏仪的应用显著增加 ROSC(比值比为 1.53,$P < 0.001$)。

参考文献:

Westfall M, Krantz S, Mullin C, Kaufman C. Mechanical versus manual chest compressions in out-of-hospital cardiac arrest. Crit Care Med 2013 Jul;41(7):1782 – 1789.

作者: **Semhar Tewelde**

心肺复苏

17. Salvage PCI and ECMO for shock-refractory ventricular fibrillation in STEMI

1. The primary goal in management of STEMI is rapid coronary revascularization. STEMI's are occasionally complicated by ventricular fibrillation (VF) arrest. High quality chest compressions and early defibrillation will improve survival. But what can be done in cases where conventional ACLS measures fail and patients have shock-refractory VF?

2. Some have suggested that emergent PCI with ongoing CPR en route may be beneficial. This option may be considered in close consultation with cardiology if the arrest is thought to be driven by ongoing ischemia and infarction. However, definitive data is lacking and this has only been described in a handful of case reports.

3. There may also be a role for venoarterial ECMO to aid in perfusion of vital organs and limit the risk of multisystem organ failure. The ECMO circuit can also help facilitate therapeutic hypothermia after the culprit vessel(s) is revascularized and rhythm is restored.

4. Chances for survival are highest in younger patients, those that do not have chronic illnesses, and those who received immediate CPR after arrest.

5. Summary: Consider emergent consultation for salvage PCI and ECMO in select cases of shock-refractory ventricular fibrillation associated with STEMI

Author: Ali Farzad

美
国
急
诊
临
床
必
知
200
招

17. 急诊 PCI 和 ECMO 在 STEMI 伴电除颤无效性室颤时的应用

1. 治疗 STEMI 的首要目标是快速冠状动脉血运重建。STEMI 偶尔会并发心室颤动（VF）心脏骤停。高质量的胸外按压和早期除颤将提高生存率。但是，在常规高级生命支持（ACLS）措施失败或患者出现除颤无效的 VF 情况下，可采取什么措施呢？

2. 有些人认为，对在转运途中进行心肺复苏的患者进行紧急 PCI 可能是有意义的。如果认为心脏骤停是由于持续缺血和梗死造成的，在与心内科医生密切磋商后，可考虑此项选择。然而，它缺乏确切的数据，也只是在极少数的病例报告中描述过。

3. VA-ECMO 在保证重要器官灌注和减少多器官衰竭风险方面可能是有作用的。在血运重建和心律恢复后还可以利用 ECMO 的管路进行低温治疗。

4. 年轻，没有慢性疾病，骤停后立即进行复苏的患者生存率是最高的。

5. 结论：在 STEMI 伴除颤无效性室颤情况下，可考虑做急诊 PCI 和 ECMO。

参考文献：

A recently published case report（attached）presents a fascinating case where salvage PCI and ECMO were used for shock-refractory VF. The patient survives with good neurological outcome. It highlights the multidisciplinary cooperation and resources necessary to utilize these heroic practices.

Brown DFM, Jaffer FA, Baker JN, Gurol ME. Case records of the Massachusetts General Hospital. Case 28 – 2013. A 52-year-old man with cardiac arrest after an acute myocardial infarction. N Engl J Med. 2013；369（11）：1047 – 1054. doi：10.1056/NEJMcpc1304164.

作者：Ali Farzad

心肺复苏

18. 2010 AHA Guidelines: procainamide is back!

1. The September 5 2006 issue of Circulation contained a guideline, based on collaboration between the American Heart Assn, the American College of Cardiology, and the European Society of Cardiology, indicating that procainamide was preferable to amiodarone for the treatment of stable monomorphic ventricular tachycardia.

2. The 2010 AHA Guidelines have now also listed procainamide as the preferred drug for stable monomorphic ventricular tachycardia, giving it a Class IIa ("probably helpful") rating vs. amiodarone which has a Class IIb ("possibly helpful") rating.

3. Procainamide is also the safest drug for use in tachydysrhythmias when an accessory pathway (e. g. Wolff-Parkinson-White syndrome) is present.

4. The caveat is that neither procainamide nor amiodarone should be used in the presence of a prolonged QTc.

5. Acute care physicians should (re-)familiarize themselves with the use of procainamide, and emergency departments should maintain quick access to this drug to stay up-to-date with current national and international guidelines.

Author: AmalMattu

18. 2010 年美国心脏病协会指南：普鲁卡因胺又回来了！

1. 2006 年 9 月 5 日由美国心脏病协会(AHA)、美国心脏病学院、欧洲心脏病学会共同在美国《循环》杂志发表了指南,指出普鲁卡因胺在治疗稳定性同型室颤时优于胺碘酮。

2. 2010 年 AHA 也将普鲁卡因胺列为在治疗稳定性同型室颤时的首选药,定位于 IIa 类(很可能有帮助),而胺碘酮则被列为 IIb 类(也许有帮助)。

3. 普鲁卡因胺也是治疗由旁路造成的快速心率失常(如预激综合征)时最安全的药。

4. 要注意的是普鲁卡因胺和胺碘酮在 QTc 延长时不要用。

5. 急诊医师要重新熟悉普鲁卡因胺的使用,根据最新的国家或国际上的指南急诊科应备有此药以便应用。

参考文献:

ACC/AHA/ESC 2006 Guidelines for Management of Patients With Ventricular Arrhythmias and the Prevention of Sudden Cardiac Death — Executive Summary (many many authors) Circulation 2006; 114: 1088 - 1132.

Neumar RW, et al. Part 8: Adult Advanced Cardiovascular Life Support: 2010 American Heart Association Guidelines for Cardiopulmonary Resuscitation and Emergency Cardiovascular Care. Circulation 2010; 122: S729 - 767.

作者: AmalMattu

心肺复苏

19. Procainamide Dosing

1. ACLS recommendation for procainamide in tachycardic rhythms is:

1) Loading dose 20 mg/minute (up to 50 mg/minute for more urgent situations) until:

(1) Arrhythmia is controlled.

(2) Hypotension occurs.

(3) QRS complex widens by 50% of its original width.

(4) total of 17 mg/kg is given.

2) Maintenance infusion is 1 to 4 mg/min.

2. An easier method for dosing acute onset atrial fibrillation in stable patients was used in the Ottawa Aggressive Protocol, in which they administered 1 gm over 60 min, which was interrupted if BP < 100 mmHg.

3. A strategy for treating stable monomorphic VT with procainamide used:

100 mg IV over 1 – 2 minutes, repeat as necessary until an endpoint of

1) Termination of tachycardia.

2) Drug induced hemodynamic deterioration.

3) Completion of 800 mg maximal dose.

4) If no slowing of the tachycardia occurred with a dose of 400 mg, the administration was ceased.

Author: Ellen Lemkin

19. 普鲁卡因胺剂量

1. ACLS 对普鲁卡因治疗心动过速的建议是：

1）负荷剂量为 20 mg/min（在更紧迫的情况下可高达 50 mg/min），直到：

（1）心律失常得到控制；

（2）出现低血压；

（3）QRS 波比基础增宽达 50%；

（4）或总剂量已达 17 mg/kg；

2）维持剂量为 1～4 mg/min。

2. 一个更简单的治疗稳定的急性心房颤动发作的给药方法是渥太华快速方案：60 分钟内给 1 g，如果血压 <100 mmHg，就要停止。

3. 用普鲁卡因胺治疗稳定的单形性室速的方案：

1～2 分钟内静脉给 100 mg，必要时可重复，直到下列任何一项出现：

1）心动过速终止；

2）药物引起的血流动力学恶化；

3）已用到 800 mg 的最大剂量；

4）如果 400 mg 后心动过速还没有慢下来，就要停止给药。

参考文献：

Steil IG, Clement CM, Perry JJ et al. Association of the Ottawa Aggressive Protocol with rapid discharge of emergency department patients with recent-onset atrial fibrillation or flutter. CJEM 2010; 12(3): 181 – 91.

Komura S, Chinushi M, Furushima H. et al. Efficacy of Procainamide and Lidocaine in Terminating Sustained Monomorphic Ventricular Tachycardia. Circulation May 2010 Vol 72

作者：**Ellen Lemkin**

心
肺
复
苏

20. Vasopressin, Steroids, and Epi···. Oh my！ A new cocktail for cardiac arrest?

1. The efficacy of epinephrine during out-of hospital cardiac arrest has been questioned in recent years, especially with respect to neurologic outcomes (ref#1).

2. A recent study demonstrated both a survival and neurologic benefit to using epinephrine during in-hospital cardiac arrest when used in combination with vasopressin and methylprednisolone.

3. Researchers in Greece randomized 268 consecutive patients with in-hospital cardiac arrest to receive either epinephrine + placebo (control group; n = 138) or vasopressin, epinephrine, and methylprednisolone (intervention arm; n = 130).

4. Vasopressin (20 IU) was given with epinephrine each CPR cycle for the first 5 cycles; Epinephrine was given alone thereafter (if necessary).

5. Methylprednisolone (40 mg) was only given during the first CPR cycle.

6. If there was return of spontaneous circulation (ROSC) but the patient was in shock, 300 mg of methylprednisolone was given daily for up to 7 days.

7. Primary study end-points were ROSC for 20 minutes or more and survival to hospital discharge while monitoring for neurological outcome.

8. The results were that patients in the intervention group had a statistically significant:

1) probability of ROSC for >20 minutes (84% vs. 66%).

2) survival with good neurological outcomes (14% vs. 5%).

3) survival if shock was present post-ROSC (21% vs. 8%).

4) better hemodynamic parameters, less organ dysfunction, and better central venous saturation levels.

9. Bottom-line: This study may present a promising new therapy for in-hospital cardiac arrest and should be strongly considered.

Author: Haney Mallemat

美
国
急
诊
临
床
必
知
200
招

20. 血管加压素、激素和肾上腺素：心脏骤停的一个新的"鸡尾酒"混合剂

1. 近几年来对肾上腺素在医院外心脏骤停的作用已有质疑，尤其是对神经系统预后的影响。

2. 最近的一项研究显示：在院内心脏骤停抢救时，当肾上腺素与血管加压素和甲泼尼龙联合使用时，可改善生存率和神经系统预后。

3. 希腊的研究人员对 268 例院内心脏骤停患者随机的分成肾上腺素 + 安慰剂组（对照组，$n = 138$）或血管加压素、肾上腺素及甲泼尼龙（治疗组，$n = 130$）。

4. 在心肺复苏的前 5 个周期，血管加压素（20 IU）与肾上腺素同时给予；然后只给肾上腺素（如果有必要的话）。

5. 甲泼尼龙（40 mg）只在第一个 CPR 周期给予。

6. 如果自主循环恢复（ROSC），但患者处于休克状态，7 天内每天要给 300 mg 的甲泼尼龙。

7. 主要终点为，ROSC 超过 20 分钟，存活出院并监测神经系统预后。

8. 结果发现，治疗组患者在下列几方面有统计学意义：

1）ROSC 恢复 > 20 分钟（84% 对 66%）；

2）神经系统恢复良好（14% 对 5%）；

3）ROSC 后出现休克的存活率（21% 比 8%）；

4）较好的血流动力学参数，较轻的器官功能障碍，和更好的中央静脉血氧饱和度水平。

9. 要点

这项研究可能会提示一个充满希望的治疗院内心脏骤停的新方法，应该引起重视。

参考文献：

Jacobs, I. et. al. Effect of adrenaline on survival in out-of-hospital cardiac arrest: A randomized double-blind placebo-controlled trial. Resuscitation 2011 Sep; 82(9): 1138 – 1143.

Spyros Mentzelopoulos et al. Vasopressin, Steroids, and Epinephrine and Neurologically Favorable Survival After In-Hospital Cardiac Arrest. A Randomized Clinical Trial. JAMA 2013; 310(3): 270 –279.

作者：Haney Mallemat

心肺复苏

21. The CORE Scan

1. The Concentrated Overview of Resuscitative Efforts (CORE) Scan

2. Ultrasound has become an essential tool in the evaluation and management of the crashing patient.

3. The CORE scan utilizes emergency bedside ultrasonography to systematically evaluate and resuscitate the rapidly deteriorating patient.

4. Essentially steps in the CORE scan include:

1) Endotracheal tube assessment

2) Lung assessment

(1) Pneumothorax?

(2) Pleural effusion?

(3) Hemothorax?

3) Cardiac assessment

(1) Pericardial effusion?

(2) Massive PE?

(3) Estimated ejection fraction?

4) Aorta assessment

(1) Abdominal aortic aneurysm?

(2) Aortic dissection?

5) IVC assessment

6) Abdominal assessment

Intraperitoneal fluid?

Author: Michael Winters

美
国
急
诊
临
床
必
知
200
招

21. 复苏措施重点评定(CORE)超声检查

1.复苏措施重点评定(CORE)超声检查。

2.超声已成为评估和抢救危重患者的重要工具。

3.CORE 超声检查利用急诊床旁超声对迅速恶化的患者进行评估以指导复苏。

4.CORE 超声检查的关键步骤包括:

1)气管插管的评估。

2)肺部评估。

(1)气胸?

(2)胸腔积液?

(3)血胸?

3)心脏评估。

(1)心包积液?

(2)严重肺栓塞?

(3)预计射血分数?

4)主动脉评估。

(1)腹主动脉瘤?

(2)主动脉夹层?

5)下腔静脉评估。

6)腹部评估。

腹腔积液。

参考文献:

Wu TS. The CORE Scan:Concentrated Overview of Resuscitative Efforts [J]. Crit Care Clin 2014;30:151-175.

作者:**Michael Winters**

心
肺
复
苏

22. To The Cath Lab-In V Fib

1. Emergency Physicians may be confronted with a case of an awake and alert patient who arrives to the ED with an acute STEMI and then develops refractory ventricular fibrillation.

2. The typical approach is to continue ACLS protocol in the ED until the V Fib is terminated, and then transfer the patient to the cardiac catheterization laboratory for emergency primary PCI.

3. However, the EP should be aware that in the setting of persistent V Fib, there is precedent for salvage PCI during ongoing CPR .

4. The interventional cardiologist may be reluctant to take the patient to the cath lab while V Fib is ongoing.

5. Since shock-refractory ventricular fibrillation in many such cases is most likely driven by ongoing ischemia and infarction, it is postulated that PCI facilitates termination of the ventricular fibrillation.

6. Advanced airway management, antiarrhythmic agents, and epinephrine or vasopressin can be given while rapidly moving the patient to revascularization in the cath lab.

7. It may be incumbent upon the EP to advocate for transfer of the patient to the cath lab in the setting of shock-refractory V Fib, especially in the setting of a patient who arrived to the ED neurologically intact.

Author: EMedHome. com

22. 要转到心导管室——在心室颤动时

1. 急诊医师可能会遇见急性 STEMI 患者，就诊时神志清楚，但随后出现顽固性心室颤动。

2. 典型的做法是在急诊科继续执行 ACLS 方案，直到心室颤动终止，然后将患者转移到心导管室行紧急 PCI。

3. 然而，急诊医生应该知道，在持续性心室颤动的情形下，有在进行心肺复苏同时进行急诊 PCI 的先例。

4. 介入心脏医生可能不愿将患者在心室颤动时送进导管室。

5. 由于除颤无反应顽固性心室颤动在许多情况下是由持续性缺血和梗死造成的，因此 PCI 有可能会有利于心室颤动的终止。

6. 有效的气道管理，抗心律失常药物，肾上腺素或血管加压素，都可以在迅速转移患者到导管室做血运重建的同时使用。

7. 提倡转移除颤无反应顽固性心室颤动患者到导管室可能是急诊医生义不容辞的责任，尤其是在到达急诊科时神经系统无异常的患者。

参考文献：

Brown DF, Jaffer FA, Baker JN, et al. Case records of the Massachusetts General Hospital. Case 28 – 2013. A 52-year-old man with cardiac arrest after an acute myocardial infarction[J]. N Engl J Med, 2013, 369: 1047 – 1054.

作者：EMedHome. com

心肺复苏

23. Keeping the Beat:
Strategies in Shock Refractory VF

Recent advances in resuscitation science have enabled emergency physicians to identify factors associated with good neurologic and survival outcomes. Cases of persistent ventricular dysrhythmia (VF or VT) present a particular challenge to the critical care provider. The evidence base for interventions in shock refractory ventricular VF mainly consists of case reports and retrospective trials, but such interventions may be worth considering in these difficult resuscitation situations:

1. Double sequential defibrillation. For shock-refractory VF, 2 sets of pads are placed (anterior/posterior and on the anterior chest wall). Shocks are delivered as "closely as possible. "

2. Sympathetic blockade in prolonged VF arrest. "Eletrical storm, " or incessant v-fib, can complicate some arrests in the setting of VF. An esmolol bolus and infusion may be associated with improved survival. Left stellate ganglion blockade has been identified as a potential treatment for medication resistant VF.

3. Don't forget about magnesium! May terminate VF due to a prolonged QT interval.

4. Invasive strategies. Though resource intensive, there is limited experience with intra-arrest PCI and extracorporeal membrane oxygenation. Preestablished protocols are key to selecting patients who may benefit from intra-arrest PCI and/or ECMO.

5. Utilization of mechanical CPR devices. Though mechanical CPR devices were not officially endorsed by the AHA/ECC 2010 guidelines, there's little question that mechanical compression devices address the complication of provider fatigue during ongoing resuscitation.

Author: Benjamin Lawner

美
国
急
诊
临
床
必
知
200
招

23. 保持心跳：顽固性室颤的新策略

复苏学的最新进展，已经能够使急诊医师明确判断具有良好的神经和生存恢复的因素。持续性的心室节律紊乱（室颤或室速）对于（急诊）危重病医生是一个特别的挑战。对电击无效的顽固性室颤治疗措施的循证基础主要来源于病例报告和回顾性试验，但在复杂的复苏情况下，这些方法还是值得考虑的：

1. 重复连续除颤。对于电击无效的顽固性心室颤动，放置 2 套除颤垫（前/后和前胸壁）。两次电击除颤越近越好。

2. 交感神经阻滞治疗延长的心室颤动骤停。"电风暴"或持续性心室颤动，增加了一些由心室颤动造成的心脏骤停的复杂程度。艾司洛尔可能会改善生存率。左侧星状神经节阻滞已被认为是对药物治疗无效心室颤动的一种潜在的治疗手段。

3. 不要忘记镁。它可能会终止由 QT 间期延长导致的心室颤动。

4. 侵入性治疗。虽然有丰富的资料，但对于骤停时进行经皮冠状动脉介入治疗和体外膜肺氧合的临床经验有限。预先设定治疗方案是选择可能受益于经皮冠状动脉介入治疗和/或体外膜肺氧合患者的关键。

5. 利用机械 CPR 装置。机械 CPR 设备虽然没有正式通过 2010 年 AHA/ECC 的认可，但有一点是没有疑问的，即机械按压设备解决了在持续复苏中医护人员疲劳的问题。

参考文献：

1. EMS World Magazine online. "Hold the coroner!" 2011. Available at：http://www. emsworld. com/article/10318805/hold-the-coroner

2. Hoch DH, Batsford WP, Greenberg SM, et al. Double sequential shocks for refractory ventricular fibrillation. J Am Coll Cardiol. 1994；23(5)：1141 – 5

3. de Oliveira FC, Feitosa-Filho GS, Ritt LE. Use of beta blockers for the treatment of cardiac arrest due to ventricular fibrillation/pulseless ventricular tachycardia：a systematic review. Resuscitation. 2012；83(6)：674 – 83

4. Patel RA, Priore DL, Szeto WY, et al, Left stellate ganglion blockade for the management of drug-resistant electrical storm. Pain medicine. 2011；12：1196 – 1198.

5. Kagawa E, Dote K, Sasaki S, et al. Should we emergently revascularize occluded coronaries for cardiac arrest? rapid response extracorporeal membrane oxygenation and intra-arrest percutaneous coronary intervention. Circulation. 2011；126(13)：1605 – 13.

作者：**Benjamin Lawner**

心肺复苏

24. Be Bold and Make Inpatients Cold

1. Therapeutic hypothermia (TH) following out-of-hospital cardiac arrest (OHCA) has increasingly been utilized since it was first described. TH following in-hospital cardiac arrest (IHCA), on the other hand, is not as commonplace or consistent despite a recommendation by the American Heart Association (AHA).

2. A recent prospective multi-center cohort-study demonstrated that of 67 498 patients with return of spontaneous circulation (ROSC) following IHCA only 2.0% of patients had TH initiated; of those 44.3% did not even achieve the target temperature (32 – 34 Celsius).

3. The factors found to be most associated with instituting TH were:

1) Younger patients;

2) Admission to non-ICU units;

3) Arrests occurring Monday through Friday (as compared to weekends);

4) Arrests within teaching hospitals (as compared to non-teaching institutions)。

4. Bottom-line: Hospitals should consider instituting and adhering to local TH protocols for in-house cardiac arrests.

Author: Haney Mallemat

24. 要积极对住院(心脏骤停)患者降温

1. 院外心脏骤停(OHCA)后的低温治疗(TH)自从提出后应用越来越广泛。相反的,尽管美国心脏协会(AHA)已有规范,但 TH 在院内心脏骤停(IHCA)的应用还不普及或标准化。

2. 一项最近发表的前瞻性多中心研究发现,在 67 498 个 IHCA 抢救后有自主循环恢复(ROSC)的患者中,只有 2.0%进行了 TH,但其中有 44.3%的患者没有达到目标体温(32~34℃)。

3. 与进行 TH 有关的因素:

1)年轻的患者;

2)收到非 ICU 病房;

3)心脏骤停发生在星期一到星期五(与周末相比);

4)心脏骤停发生在教学医院(与非教学医院相比)。

4. 结论:医院要对院内心脏骤停患者严格按照实施方案进行 TH。

参考文献:

Mikkelsen, M. et al. Use of Therapeutic Hypothermia After In-Hospital Cardiac Arrest. Crit Care Med 2013 Jun; 41(6): 1385 – 1395

作者: **Haney Mallemat**

心肺复苏

25. ACLS for Left Ventricular Assist Devices (LVAD) patients

1. Basics for an LVAD

1) Indications for an LVAD: Extreme left-sided heart failure awaiting a transplant and reversible heart disease such as myocarditis.

2) LVAD is temporary until disease reverses then it will be removed.

3) LVAD is permanent as patient is not a candidate for transplant.

2. ACLS for LVAD patients

1) First should assess if the LVAD is functioning

(1) Check the battery to make sure it is charged.

(2) Checking a pulse is not reliable as a pulse may not be palpable.

(3) Get a manual BP cuff and find MAP or listen for a hum.

①If a MAP or hum is present, treat as such with fluids, vasopressors, etc.

②If no MAP or hum is present, should perform CPR.

2) CPR is controversial

(1) Manufacturers manual recommends no CPR for fear of dislodging the device and leaving a gaping hole in the heart.

(2) However, the patient is dead if the device is not working and the heart is not pumping so CPR is at least attempting to resuscitate.

3) Defibrillation/Cardioversion

(1) Acceptable to shock hearts with LVADs.

(2) Be sure to disconnect from the power source prior to shocking.

Authors: Haney Mallemat, MD and Michael Winters, MD

25.左心室辅助装置(LVAD)患者的 ACLS

1.什么是 LVAD

1)LVAD 的指征:等待移植的极度左心力衰竭和可逆性心脏病,如心肌炎。

2)LVAD 是临时的,可在疾病纠正后撤掉。

3)如患者不适合做移植,LVAD 将是永久的。

2.LVAD 患者如何实施 ACLS

1)首先要判断 LVAD 是否工作正常

(1)检查电池是否有电;

(2)检查脉搏是不可靠的,因为可能摸不到;

(3)手工量一下血压,寻找"哼"音;

①如果有血压和哼音,给液体,升压药等;

②如没有血压或哼音,做 CPR。

2)CPR 是有争议的

(1)厂商说明书不建议做 CPR,考虑到它有可能使仪器脱节,在心脏上留下一个洞。

(2)但如果 LVAD 不工作,心脏就不跳动,患者就死了。CPR 至少可以试着用来复苏。

3)除颤/转复。

(1)可以电击 LVAD 的心脏;

(2)一定要在电击前切断电源。

参考文献:

1. Rose EA, Gellins AC, Moskovitz AJ, et al. Long-Term Use of a Left Ventricular Assist Device for End-Stage Heart Failure. NEJM. 2001; 345(20): 1435 - 43.

2. Wilson SR, et al. Ventricular assist devices. JACC. 2009; 54(18): 1647 - 59.

3. Klein T, Jacob MS. Management of implantable assisted circulation devices. Cardiol Clin. 2012; 30: 673 - 82.

作者:**Haney Mallemat, MD and Michael Winters, MD**

心肺复苏

26. Coronary Angiography in Out-of-Hospital-Cardiac-Arrest（OHCA）

1. Acute coronary thrombotic occlusion is the most common trigger of cardiac arrest.

2. The benefit of coronary angiography seems to be well established in patients who regain consciousness soon after recovery of spontaneous circulation（ROSC）.

3. Whether emergency coronary angiography and PCI improve survival in patients who remain unconscious after ROSC remains unknown.

4. Results of this study can be summarized as follows：

1）CAD and acute or recent culprit coronary lesions are present in most resuscitated unconscious patients with OHCA without obvious extracardiac cause.

2）CAD and acute or recent culprit coronary lesions are observed in most patients with ST-segment elevation and in a non-negligible proportion of patients with other ECG patterns on post-ROSC electrocardiograph.

3）Emergency coronary angiography and successful emergency PCI are independently related to in-hospital survival after OHCA.

Author：Semhar Tewelde

美
国
急
诊
临
床
必
知
200
招

26. 冠状动脉造影在院外心脏骤停 (OHCA) 中的应用

1. 急性冠状动脉血栓栓塞是心脏骤停最常见的诱发因素。

2. 冠状动脉造影对自主循环恢复(ROSC)后很快清醒患者的应用价值好像是成立的。

3. 但是，紧急冠状动脉造影和经皮冠状动脉介入能否改善 ROSC 后意识没有恢复患者的预后还不清楚。

4. 这个临床研究结果可以归纳为如下几点：

1) 多数 OHCA 复苏后神志不清且没有明显心脏以外原因的患者可发现有冠心病和急性或新近发生的冠状动脉病变。

2) 多数有 ST 段抬高和相当一部分 ROSC 后有不可忽略心电图变化的患者可发现有冠心病和急性或新近发生的冠状动脉病变。

3) 紧急冠状动脉造影和成功的急诊 PCI 与改善 OHCA 后住院生存率有独立的关系。

参考文献：

Zanuttini D, Armellini I, et al. Impact of Emergency Coronary Angiography on In-Hospital Outcome of Unconscious Survivors After Out-of-Hospital Cardiac Arrest Original. J Am Coll Cardiol 2012；110：12 pages 1723 – 1728.

作者：**Semhar Tewelde**

27. Post – Arrest Syndrome

1. Goal of post-arrest syndrome care is to mitigate:

1) Injury to brain.

2) Injury to heart.

3) Inflammatory mediators.

2. Initiate therapeutic hypothermia (neuroprotective)

3. Definitively control airway

1) Intubate now if not already done during the code.

2) Avoid hyperventilation.

3) Avoid hyperoxia (goal O_2 saturation in low 90 s).

4. Manage blood pressure

1) Invasive hemodynamic monitoring (arterial line) preferred.

2) Goal MAP 80 – 90.

3) May require vasopressors.

4) Critically important to avoid episodes of hypotension.

5. Treat underlying cause of arrest

If presumed cardiac cause, need to send patient to cath lab

(1) Can still cool prior to/during cath lab.

(2) 2013 STEMI guidelines consider it a Class I indication to cool and cath a post-arrest patient that has STEMI on ECG

6. Sedation & paralysis

1) Shivering increases metabolic demand and heat production.

2) If shivering, paralyze.

3) Benzodiazepines can also help prevent shivering.

7. Seizure control

1) Consider non-convulsive status, particularly if patient paralyzed.

2) Consider continuous EEG.

3) Liberal use of benzodiazepines or propofol can help prevent; not enough literature to support prophylactic anti-epileptics.

4) If see seizure activity, treat aggressively.

8. Glucose control

1) Keep glucose in a "normal" range.

Probably "tight" glucose control is not necessary.

2) Unclear what ideal numbers are.

9. Prophylactic antibiotics

Aspiration is very common, but aggressive empiric antibiotics not of benefit unless evidence of aspiration pneumonia on x-ray or clinically.

10. Steroids

1) No evidence to support routine use.

2) Reasonable if regractory hypotention or history suggestive of adrenal insufficiency.

11. Renal replacement therapy?

1) No routine role for dialysis.

2) Monitor electrolytes & urine output.

12. Bottom Line

1) Keep MAP > 80, & monitor end-organ perfusion.

2) Initiate therapeutic hypothermia.

3) Send to the cath lab if potential cardiac cause of arrest.

Author: Ben Lawner

心
肺
复
苏

57

27. 心脏骤停后综合征

1. 治疗心脏骤停后综合征的目的是减轻：

1）脑损伤；

2）心脏损伤；

3）炎症反应。

2. 应用治疗性低温（神经保护）

3. 完全控制呼吸道

1）如在抢救时没有插管，进行插管；

2）避免过度通气；

3）避免过度给氧（保持氧饱和度在刚过 90%）。

4. 控制血压

1）最好放置动脉导管以监测血液动力学指标；

2）理想平均动脉压为 80 ~ 90 mmHg；

3）可使用升压药；

4）防止低血压的发生是非常重要的。

5. 治疗造成心脏骤停的原因

如考虑是心脏方面的原因，要将患者送到导管室。

（1）在导管前或导管中都要保持低温；

（2）2013 年 STEMI 指南将低温和导管治疗列为 ECG 显示 STEMI 的心脏骤停后患者的推荐方案（closs I）。

6. 镇静和肌肉松弛

1）颤抖会增加代谢和热的产生；

2）一旦有颤抖，就要给肌松药；

3）苯二氮䓬类可帮助防止颤抖。

7. 癫痫的控制

1）如患者处于瘫痪状态，要考虑非惊厥性癫痫的可能；

2）要考虑做脑电图；

3）苯二氮䓬类和丙泊酚的适量使用会起到预防作用；没有文献支持抗癫痫预防性用药；

4）一旦发现癫痫发作，要积极处理。

8. 血糖控制

1）保持血糖在正常范围，不需要"严格"控制血糖；

2）理想的范围还不清楚。

9. 预防性使用抗生素？

误吸是非常常见的，但如胸片或临床上没有吸入性肺炎的征象，积极使用抗生素没有益处

10. 激素

1）没有证据支持激素的常规使用；

2）在顽固性低血压或有肾上腺功能低下病史时，可考虑使用。

11. 肾脏替代治疗

1）不需要常规使用透析；

2）监测电解质和尿量。

12. 要点

1）维持 MAP > 80 mmHg，监测各器官灌注

2）进行治疗性低温

3）如由心脏的原因引起，送导管室

参考文献：

Reynolds JC, Lawner BJ. Management of the post-cardiac arrest syndrome. Journal of Emergency Medicine 2012；42：440 – 449.

作者：Ben Lawner

28. Capnography in finding the causes of cardiac arrest

1. Review of capnography

1)2010 European Resuscitation Council recommended using waveform capnography during cardiac arrest to guide CPR.

2)2010 AHA guidelines made it a Class 2B recommendation.

2. Uses for capnography

1) Has a specificity of 97 – 100% for confirming correct placement of endotracheal tube.

2) Useful for CPR.

If < 10 mmHg, it may be that CPR is inadequate and providers should maximize effectiveness of compressions by switching out or pushing harder.

3) Useful for alerting providers there is a return of spontaneous circulation (ROSC).

(1) If end-tidal CO_2 ($ETCO_2$) is 30 – 40, has positive correlation with ROSC.

(2) If there is a sudden increase of 15 – 25 above the baseline $ETCO_2$, also has a positive correlation with ROSC.

(3) This can help minimize interruptions in compressions for pulse check.

3. If $ETCO_2$ is persistently < 10 mmHg for 20 minutes despite adequate CPR, chances of ROSC are slim

4. Use of $ETCO_2$ for determining the cause of arrest – Resuscitation article

1) Respiratory arrest patients had higher mean $ETCO_2$ (in the mid 20's mmHg) compared to other causes. Thought to be from retained CO_2 from diminished ventilation.

2) Pulmonary embolus patients had lower mean $ETCO_2$ than cardiac arrest and respiratory arrest. Thought to be due to decreased pulmonary blood flow and increased alveolar dead space.

3) Patients who had eventual ROSC had higher initial $ETCO_2$ compared to patients who did not have ROSC.

Author: John Greenwood, MD

美
国
急
诊
临
床
必
知
200
招

28. 二氧化碳描记图及其在鉴定骤停原因时的应用

1. 二氧化碳描记图简介

1)2010 年欧洲复苏委员会建议在心脏骤停抢救中使用波形式二氧化碳描记图指导 CPR；

2)2010 年美国心脏协会指南把它列为推荐类别 2B。

2. 二氧化碳描记图的使用

1)在确定气管内插管正确位置方面的特异性达 97% ~ 100%；

2)在 CPR 时非常有用

如低于 10 mmHg，说明 CPR 效果差，需要通过换人或更有力地按压以达到最大按压效果

3)在自主循环恢复(ROSC)时可发出示警。

(1)如呼吸末期 CO_2($ETCO_2$)为 30 ~ 40 mmHg，与 ROSC 有明确的关系。

(2)如果 $ETCO_2$ 突然比基线升高 15 ~ 20 mmHg，同样预示着 ROSC。

(3)它有助于最大限度地减少因检查脉搏而中断按压。

3. 即使 CPR 有效，如 $ETCO_2$ 持续 20 min 低于 10 mmHg，标志着 ROSC 的机会非常小

4. 用 $ETCO_2$ 确定心脏骤停的原因(复苏杂志的文章)

1)与其他原因比较，呼吸性骤停的患者会有较高的 $ETCO_2$(约 25 mmHg)。这可能是由低通气造成的 CO_2 储留。

2)与心脏和呼吸骤停相比，肺动脉栓塞患者的 $ETCO_2$ 较低，可能是由肺动脉血流减低和肺泡死腔增加造成的。

3)ROSC 患者的 $ETCO_2$ 要比没有 ROSC 的患者要高。

参考文献：

Heradstveit BE, Sunde K, et al. Factors complicating interpretation of capnography during advanced life support in cardiac arrest-a clinical retrospective study in 575 patients. Resuscitation. 2012 Jul;83(7):813 –818.

作者：**John Greenwood，MD**

心肺复苏

心脏病
Cardiology

29. 2013 ACCF/AHA Guideline for the Management of ST Elevation Myocardial Infarction (part 1, System and PCI)?

Regional system and Primary percutaneous coronary intervention (PCI)

1. Performance of a 12-lead electrocardiogram (ECG) by emergency medical services personnel at the site of first medical contact (FMC) is recommended in patients with symptoms consistent with STEMI.

2. Reperfusion therapy should be administered to all eligible patients with STEMI with symptom onset within the prior 12 hours.

3. Primary PCI is the recommended method of reperfusion when it can be performed in a timely fashion by experienced operators.

4. Emergency medical services transport directly to a PCI-capable hospital for primary PCI is the recommended triage strategy for patients with STEMI, with an ideal FMC-to-device time system goal of 90 minutes or less.

5. Immediate transfer to a PCI-capable hospital for primary PCI is the recommended triage strategy for patients with STEMI who initially arrive at or are transported to a non-PCI-capable hospital, with an FMC-to-device time system goal of 120 minutes or less.

6. In the absence of contraindications, fibrinolytic therapy should be administered to patients with STEMI at non-PCI-capable hospitals when the anticipated FMC-to-device time at a PCI-capable hospital exceeds 120 minutes because of unavoidable delays.

7. When fibrinolytic therapy is indicated or chosen as the primary reperfusion strategy, it should be administered within 30 minutes of hospital arrival.

8. Reperfusion therapy is reasonable for patients with STEMI and symptom onset within the prior 12 to 24 hours who have clinical and/or ECG evidence of ongoing ischemia. Primary PCI is the preferred strategy in this population.

9. Primary PCI should be performed in patients with STEMI and cardiogenic shock or acute severe HF, irrespective of time delay from myocardial infarction (MI) onset.

Author: Feng Xiao

29. 2013 年美国心脏病学会基金会(ACCF)和美国心脏病协会(AHA)ST 段抬高心肌梗死(STEMI)治疗指南(第一部分:医疗系统和 PCI)

区域医疗系统和早期经皮冠状动脉介入治疗:

1. 紧急医疗服务人员在现场第一时间内对怀疑 STEMI 的患者做 12 导联心电图。

2. 在症状出现后 12 h 内对所有 STEMI 患者进行再灌注治疗。

3. 由有具有经验的操作者尽快进行早期经皮冠状动脉介入治疗(PCI)。

4. EMS 要在 90 min 内将 STEMI 患者从第一现场直接送到具有 PCI 能力的医院的 PCI 设备旁。

5. 如果 STEMI 患者就诊于或被送到一个不能做 PCI 的医院,要在 120 min 内迅速地将患者转运到能做 PCI 的医院。

6. 在没有禁忌证的情况下,对于在不能做 PCI 的医院或由于不可避免的延误造成不能在 120 min 内将 STEMI 患者转到有 PCI 能力的医院的,要进行溶栓治疗。

7. 如果溶栓治疗作为首选再灌注手段,要在患者到达医院 30 min 内开始。

8. 在 12 ~ 24 h 内,如 STEMI 患者有临床和/或 ECG 持续缺血表现,也可以进行再灌注治疗。PCI 也是首选的。

9. 对于合并有心源性休克或急性严重心力衰竭的 STEMI 患者,不论从发病开始所耽误的时间有多长,都要进行早期 PCI。

参考文献:

J Am Coll Cardiol. 2013;61(4):485 – 510.

作者: **Feng Xiao** 肖锋

心脏病

30. 2013 ACCF/AHA Guideline for the Management of ST Elevation Myocardial Infarction (part 2, routine medical therapies)?

Routine Medical Therapies

1. Aspirin

Aspirin 162 to 325 mg should be given before primary PCI. After PCI, aspirin should be continued indefinitely.

2. P2Y12 receptor inhibitors

A loading dose of a P2Y12 receptor inhibitor should be given as early as possible or at time of primary PCI to patients with STEMI. Options include clopidogrel 600 mg or prasugrel 60 mg or ticagrelor 180 mg.

P2Y12 inhibitor therapy should be given for 1 year to patients with STEMI who receive a stent (bare-metal or drug-eluting) during primary PCI using the following maintenance doses: clopidogrel 75 mg daily or prasugrel 10 mg daily or ticagrelor 90 mg twice a day.

3. Anticoagulants

For patients with STEMI undergoing primary PCI, the following supportive anticoagulant regimens are recommended: UFH, taking into account whether a GP IIb/IIIa receptor antagonist has been administered; or Bivalirudin with or without prior treatment with UFH.

4. Beta blockers

Oral beta blockers should be initiated in the first 24 hours in patients with STEMI who do not have any of the following: signs of HF, evidence of a low-output state, increased risk for cardiogenic shock, or other contraindications to use of oral beta blockers (PR interval more than 0.24 seconds, second- or third-degree heart block, active asthma, or reactive airways disease).

It is reasonable to administer intravenous beta blockers at the time of presentation to patients with STEMI and no contraindications to their use who are hypertensive or have ongoing ischemia.

5. Angiotensin-converting enzyme inhibitors

An angiotensin-converting enzyme inhibitor should be administered within the first 24 hours to all patients with STEMI with anterior location, HF, or ejection fraction less than or equal to 0.40, unless contraindicated.

An angiotensin receptor blocker should be given to patients with STEMI who have indications for but are intolerant of angiotensin-converting enzyme inhibitors

6. Aldosterone antagonists

An aldosterone antagonist should be given to patients with STEMI and no contraindications who are already receiving an angiotensin-converting enzyme inhibitor and beta blocker and who have an ejection fraction less than or equal to 0.40 and either symptomatic HF or diabetes mellitus.

7. High-intensity statins

High-intensity statin therapy should be initiated or continued in all patients with STEMI and no contraindications to its use.

Author: Feng Xiao

心
脏
病

30. 2013 年 ACCF 和 AHA ST 段抬高心肌梗死(STEMI)治疗指南 (第二部分: 常规药物治疗)

常规药物治疗

1. 阿司匹林

要在 PCI 前给予 162~325 mg 阿司匹林。PCI 后需永久服用阿司匹林。

2. P2Y12 受体抑制药

尽快或在对 STEMI 患者进行 PCI 时给予负荷量的 P2Y12 受体抑制药,如氯吡格雷 600 mg 或普拉格雷 60 mg 或替卡格雷 180 mg。

对通过 PCI 接受支架(裸金属或药物涂层)治疗的 STEMI 患者,要用 1 年的 P2Y12 受体抑制剂,其维持剂量为氯吡格雷 75 mg 每天一次或普拉格雷 10 mg 每天一次或替卡格雷 90 mg 每天两次。

3. 抗凝剂

对接受 PCI 的 STEMI 患者,建议应用如下抗凝方案:普通肝素,要考虑 GPI-Ib/IIIa 受体拮抗药;或比伐芦丁(不管患者在此前是否用过普通肝素)。

4. β 受体阻滞药

STEMI 的患者只要没有下列情况,都应在 24 h 内口服 β 受体阻滞药:心力衰竭体征,低心输出量,心源性休克的可能性增加,或其他口服 β 受体阻滞药的禁忌证(PR 间期超过 0.24 s,2 或 3 度传导阻滞,哮喘发作或反应性呼吸道疾病)。

对没有禁忌证但血压高或有持续性缺血的 STEMI 患者,在就诊时可以考虑静脉给 β 受体阻滞药。

5. 血管紧张素转换酶抑制药

前壁心肌梗死、心力衰竭、或射血分数等于或低于 0.40 的 STEMI 患者在 24 h 内要给血管紧张素转换酶抑制药,除非有禁忌证。

如 STEMI 患者有如上指征,但不能耐受血管紧张素转换酶抑制药时,可用血管紧张素受体拮抗药。

6. 醛固酮拮抗药

对于已经在用血管紧张素转换酶抑制药和 β 受体阻滞药,心搏指数仍等于或低于 0.40，并有心力衰竭的表现或糖尿病的 STEMI 患者，如无禁忌证，要用醛固酮拮抗药。

7. 大剂量他汀类药物

只要没有禁忌证，大剂量他汀类药物要应用于所有的 STEMI 患者。

参考文献：

J Am Coll Cardiol. 2013；61（4）：485－510.

作者：**Feng Xiao** 肖锋

心
脏
病

31. Optimal Timing of Coronary Invasive Strategy in NSTEMI

1. International guidelines recommend early invasive strategy (< 24hrs) for patients with NSTEMI w/high risk factors defined by a GRACE score > 140.

2. A recent meta-analysis based on 7 RCTs & 4 observational studies demonstrated an inconclusive survival benefit with an early invasive strategy.

3. Heterogeneity across multiple studies including timing of intervention, definition of MI, patients' risk profiles, major bleeding, and sample size make the interpretation of survival results difficult.

4. Based on the most recent data the optimal timing of intervention remains unclear and a more definite RCT is warranted to guide clinical practice.

Author: Semhar Tewelde

31. 对非 ST 段抬高心肌梗死(NSTEMI) 冠状动脉介入治疗措施的最佳时间

1. 国际指南建议对 GRACE 评分超过 140 的高危险 NSTEMI 患者,要早期进行介入治疗(24 h 内)。

2. 一项最新的对 7 个随机对照研究和 4 个观察性研究的 meta 分析显示,早期介入治疗并不能明确地改善预后。

3. 这些研究在治疗时间,心肌梗死的定义,患者的危险因素,大出血和样本量的不一致性给生存率的分析造成了困难。

4. 依据最新的资料,介入治疗的最佳时间还不明了,需要一个相当明确的随机对照研究来指导临床实践。

参考文献:

Navarese E, et al. Optimal Timing of Coronary Invasive Strategy in Non-ST-Segment Elevation A-cute Coronary Syndromes. Ann Intern Med. 2013; 158: 261 – 270.

作者: Semhar Tewelde

心脏病

32. AMI dianostic Criteria：Sgarbossa Criteria

1. Sgarbossa et al, initially identified patients with MI and left bunde branch block (LBBB) from the GUSTO trial; these ECGs were compared to the ECGs of patients with chronic CAD and LBBB.

2. LBBB is defined by 3 criteria QRS >125 ms, V1 – QS or rS, and R wave peak time 60ms with no q wave in leads I, V5, V6.

3. After a criteria to identify MI with LBBB was estabilshed it was tested on patients presenting with chest pain and LBBB.

4. The study resulted in Sgarbossa criteria; 3 independent predictors of MI in setting of LBBB.

1) ST segment concordance of 1 mm any lead (greatest odd ratio, i. e. most specific).

2) ST depression 1 mm V1 – V3.

3) Excessive ST discordance greater than 5mm (lowest odds ratio).

Author：Dan Lemkin

32. 心肌梗死诊断标准：Sgarbossa 标准

1. Sgarbossa 等人首先在 GUSTO 临床研究中时有心肌梗死和左束支传导阻滞（LBBB）的患者进行研究，并将他们的心电图和具有慢性冠心病和 LBBB 的患者的心电图进行了比较。

2. LBBB 的 3 个诊断标准为：QRS > 125 ms，V1 导联呈 QS 或 rS，R 波高峰时间 > 60 ms 并且在 I，V5，V6 导联没有 q 波。

3. 在确定了诊断急性心肌梗死伴 LBBB 的诊断标准后，将此标准在具有 LBBB 的心绞痛患者中进行临床研究。

4. Sgarbossa 标准由此产生：即 3 个相互独立的 LBBB 患者急性心肌梗死的预测因素。

1）在任何导联里，同向 ST 段抬高超过 1 mm（比值比最高，即最特异）；

2）V1 – V3 ST 导联段降低超过 1 mm；

3）相反方向的 ST 抬高或降低超过 5 mm（比值比最低，相关性较低）。

参考文献：

Sgarbossa E, et al. Electrocardiographic diagnosis of evolving acute myocardial infarction in the presence of left bundle-branch block. NEJM Feb 22, 1996；Vol 334；No. 8.

作者：**Dan Lemkin**

心
脏
病

33. Third Universal Definition of MI

Type 1: Ischemic myocardial necrosis secondary to plaque rupture (ACS).

Type 2: Ischemic myocardial necrosis not secondary to ACS, but rather supply/demand mismatch, vasospasm, emboli, anemia, hypoperfusion, and/or arrhythmia.

Type 3: Sudden cardiac death.

Type 4a: PCI related.

Type 4b: Stent thrombosis.

Type 5: CABG related.

Author: Semhar Tewelde

33. 2012 年第 3 版心肌梗死通用定义

1 型：由于冠状动脉硬化斑块破裂造成的缺血性心肌坏死（急性冠状动脉综合征，ACS）。

2 型：不是由 ACS 造成的缺血性心肌坏死，如血供与需求失衡、血管痉挛、栓塞、贫血、低灌注和（或）心律紊乱。

3 型：突发性心脏骤停。

4 型 a：与经皮冠状动脉介入治疗相关的。

4 型 b：支架血栓形成。

5 型：与冠状动脉搭桥术有关的。

参考文献：

Thygesen K, Alpert JS, Jaffe AS, et al. Third universal definition of myocardial infarction. J Am Coll Cardiol 2012；60：1581 – 1598

作者：Semhar Tewelde

心
脏
病

34. Troponinonly in diagnosing patients within 2 hours of chest pain

1. The ADAPT (2-Hour Accelerated Diagnostic Protocol to Assess Patients With Chest Pain Symptoms Using Contemporary Troponins as the Only Biomarker) trial was a prospective observational validation study designed to assess a predefined ADP (Accelerated Diagnostic Protocol).

2. A low risk patient in this ADP was defined by TIMI 0, ECG w/no ischemic changes, and negative troponin at 0-and 2-hours after presentation.

3. Primary endpoint was assessment of any major adverse cardiac event (MACE).

4. Of 1, 975 patients enrolled, 302 (15.3%) had a MACE.

5. ADP classified 392 patients (20%) as low risk and only 1 (0.25%) had a MACE.

6. ADP had a sen 99.7%, NPV 99.7%, spec 23.4%, and PPV 19.0%.

7. ADP still requires rapid early outpatient follow-up or further inpatient testing.

Author: Semhar Tewelde

34. 仅用肌钙蛋白在 2 h 内
评价胸痛患者价值的研究

1. ADAPT(应用目前心肌肌钙蛋白作为唯一的生物指标来评估具有胸痛的患者)是一项前瞻性的观察性的论证临床研究,其目的是对一个快速诊断方案(ADP)进行评估。

2. ADP 中所指的低危险患者是指在就诊时和就诊 2 h 后 TIMI 为 0,没有缺血性 ECG 改变,肌钙蛋白阴性。

3. 主要观察指标是对任何的显著不良心脏后果(MACE)进行分析。

4. 在 1975 位患者中,有 302(15.3%)位患者出现 1 个 MACE。

5. 在 392 位 ADP 认定的低危险患者(20%)中,仅有 1 位患者(0.25%)有 1个 MACE 发生。

6. ADP 的敏感性为 99.7%,阴性预测值 99.7%,特异性 23.4%,阳性预测值 19.0%。

7. ADP 方案还是需要快速早期的院外随诊或进一步的院内检查。

参考文献:

Than M, Cullen L. 2-Hour Accelerated Diagnostic Protocol to Assess Patients With Chest Pain Symptoms Using Contemporary Troponins as the Only Biomarker. J Am Coll Cardiol. 2012; 59(23): 2091 – 2098

作者: **Semhar Tewelde**

心脏病

35. Troponin revisit in 2012?

1. Background

1) No real robust data exists on the interpretation of elevated troponins.

2) Elevated troponins can be difficult to interpret but are often assumed to equal acute coronary syndrome (ACS).

3) History

(1) Troponins began being used in the 1990's.

(2) There are now new ultra-sensitive assays that are meant to be faster and more sensitive for diagnosing ACS.

(3) Remember that troponin is just a laboratory marker that indicates myocardial necrosis, not necessarily myocardial infarction.

2. Interpretation and use of troponins

1) Most important parts of evaluating for ACS

(1) History of present illness.

(2) EKG.

(3) TIMI risk factors.

2) Clinical scenarios

(1) If patient has presumed ACS and elevated troponin but no ECG changes, they should not go to the cath lab unless there is a rise in troponins >20%.

(2) Patient with PE, even with RV dysfunction, troponins are not necessary.

(3) CHF patients likely have a baseline elevated troponin so should trend troponins instead of relying on one elevated value.

(4) Chronic kidney disease patients also likely have a baseline elevated troponin so should trend troponins.

(5) Sepsis patients likely have elevated troponins from LV dysfunction, increased oxygen demand, and hypoperfusion.

(6) Pericarditis and myocarditis usually have elevated troponin from inflammation instead of ischemia.

(7) All of these scenarios warrant troponin trending.

3) How to trend troponin

Next set of troponins should be greater than 3 standard deviations away from the initial set in 3 – 6 hours.

Author: Semhar Tewelde

心
脏
病

35. 2012 年对肌钙蛋白的认识

1. 背景

1) 对肌钙蛋白增高的解释，没有绝对的标准；

2) 增高的肌钙蛋白的意义是很难确定的，但通常用来确诊急性冠状动脉综合征(ACS)。

2. 历史

1) 肌钙蛋白的使用始于 19 世纪 90 年代；

2) 现在有超敏感分析方法，主要是为了更快和更敏感地诊断 ACS；

3) 要记住，肌钙蛋白只是一个标志心肌坏死的实验室指标，与心肌梗死无必然的联系。

3. 肌钙蛋白的解释和应用

1) 诊断 ACS 最主要的指标

(1) 现病史；

(2) 心电图；

(3) TIMI 危险因素。

2) 临床表现

(1) 如怀疑有 ACS 的患者肌钙蛋白水平升高，但没有 ECG 的变化，不要将他们转到导管室，除非肌钙蛋白水平的升高超过20%；

(2) 肺梗塞的患者，即使有右心力衰竭，检测肌钙蛋白也不是必要的；

(3) 慢性心力衰竭的患者常有肌钙蛋白基础水平增高，因此需要看它的趋势而不是依赖某一个点的值；

(4) 慢性肾衰的患者的基础肌钙蛋白的水平也常增高，要参考增高趋势；

(5) 败血症的患者由于左心力衰竭，氧耗量增加和低灌注而常有肌钙蛋白增高；

(6) 心包炎和心肌炎也常由于炎症而不是缺血造成肌钙蛋白增高；

(7) 在所有这些情况下，都要考虑肌钙蛋白增高趋势。

3) 如何判断肌钙蛋白增高趋势

在 3~6 h 内，肌钙蛋白的增加超过基础水平的 3 个标准差。

参考文献：

Newby LK, Jesse RL, et al. ACCF 2012 Expert Consensus Document on practical clinical considerations in the interpretation of troponin elevations: a report of the American College of Cardiology Foundation Task Force on Clinical Expert Consensus Documents. J Am Coll Cardiol. 2012; 60(23): 2427-2463.

作者: Semhar Tewelde

36. Left Ventricular Hypertrophy and STEMI

1. Identifying ST-segment changes in patients with LVH is frequently associated with false-positive diagnoses of acute coronary syndrome.

2. This study analyzed the ACTIVATE-SF database, a registry of consecutive emergency department STEMI diagnoses from 2 medical centers (411 patients).

3. In patients with anterior territory ST-elevation, using a ratio of ST segment to R-S-wave magnitude >25% as a diagnostic criteria for STEMI significantly improved specificity for an angiographic culprit lesion (true positive).

4. Although this rule requires further study in a larger population it may augment current criteria for determining which patients with ECG LVH should undergo PCI.

Author: Semhar Tewelde

36. 左心室肥厚(LVH)
与 ST 段抬高心肌梗死(STEMI)

1. 根据 ST 段变化诊断 LVH 患者是否有急性冠脉综合征时,往往会出现假阳性。

2. 本研究分析了 ACTIVATE-SF 数据库,记录了从 2 个医疗中心(411 例)的急诊科就诊的全部 STEMI 患者。

3. 对于前壁 ST 段抬高患者,用 ST 段与 R – S 波高度比值大于25% 作为 STEMI 的诊断标准可明显提高阳性血管造影的特异性(真阳性)。

4. 虽然这条规则还需要在更大的人群中做进一步的研究,但它会强化现有的诊断标准,以确定哪些心电图有 LVH 变化的患者需要经皮冠状动脉介入治疗。

参考文献:

Armstrong E, Kulkarni A, et al. Electrocardiographic Criteria for ST-Elevation Myocardial Infarction in Patients With Left Ventricular Hypertrophy. Am J Cardiol 2012; 110: 977 – 983.

作者: **Semhar Tewelde**

心脏病

37. Is RBBB More Indicative
of Large Anteroseptal MI?

1. Conventionally a new onset left bundle branch (LBBB) with acute myocardial infarction (MI) is associated with a massive MI.

2. Proximal left anterior descending artery (LAD) septal perforators perfuse the right bundle branch and the anterior fascicle of the left bundle branch ~90% of cases.

3. The right coronary artery (RCA) perfuses the posterior fascicle of the left bundle branch ~90% of cases.

4. Given the anatomy, a LAD occlusion should cause RBBB and/or LAFB; both a proximal LAD and RCA occlusion would be required for MI to cause LBBB.

5. A recent cohort study analyzed 233 patients to evaluate if RBBB or LBBB was associated with a large anteroseptal scar:

1) RBBB was associated with larger scar size (24% vs. 6.5%; $P < 0.0001$).

2) RBBB was more indicative of ischemic heart disease (79% vs. 29%; $P < 0.0001$).

6. Based on this preliminary data RBBB may have a stronger association with ischemia and anteroseptal scarring than LBBB (* limitations -small cohort of cardiomyopathy patients with an EF < 35%, further study is required).

Author: Semhar Tewelde

37. 右束支传导阻滞更能提示大面积前间壁心肌梗死吗？

1. 传统认为心肌梗死后新发生的左束支传导阻滞(LBBB)与大面积心肌梗死(MI)有关。

2. 90%的病例中，左前降支近端(LAD)的室间隔支灌注右束支和左束支的前分支。

3. 90%的病例中，右冠状动脉(RCA)灌注左束支的后分支。

4. 从解剖意义上讲，LAD 闭塞将导致右束支传导阻滞和/或左前降支(LAFB)阻滞；要造成左束支传导阻滞则需要近端 LAD 和 RCA 都闭塞。

5. 最近的一项队列研究对 233 例患者进行分析，以评估右束支传导阻滞还是左束支传导阻滞与大面积前间壁疤痕有关：

1) 右束支传导阻滞与较大的疤痕相关(24% vs 6.5%，$P < 0.0001$)

2) 右束支传导阻滞在预测缺血性心脏疾病时更有意义(79% vs 29%，$P < 0.0001$)

6. 基于这一前期数据，RBBB 与前间壁缺血和疤痕的关系要比左束支传导阻滞强(局限性：心肌病患者伴 EF < 35% 的小队列研究，需要进一步证实)。

参考文献：

Strauss DG, Loring Z, Selvester RH, et al. Right, But Not Left, Bundle Branch Block Is Associated With Large Anteroseptal Scar[J]. JACC, 2013, 62(11)：959 – 967.

作者：**Semhar Tewelde**

心脏病

38. Loss of Precordial T-Wave Balance

1. Typically the normal ECG shows progression of T-wave size across the precordial leads & the T-wave in V1 is inverted or flat.

2. A large upright T-wave in V1 can be considered normal when there is high voltage/LVH or LBBB.

3. A new upright T-wave in V1 can be indicative of significant atherosclerotic disease.

4. If the T-wave in V1 is larger than the T-wave in V6 have a high suspicion for myocardial disease.

5. A new tall upright T-wave in V1 has ~84% specificity for ischemic heart disease (Barthwal).

Author: Semhar Tewelde

38. 胸前导联 T 波异常

1. 通常情况下，正常的心电图胸前导联 T 波应该是逐渐增高，V1 的 T 波应倒置或平坦。

2. 当有高电压/左室肥厚或左束支传导阻滞时，V1 导联高大直立 T 波可以认为是正常的。

3. 一个新出现的 V1 导联直立 T 波，标志着动脉粥样硬化性疾病。

4. 如果 V1 导联 T 波大于 V6 导联，要高度怀疑心肌病。

5. 在 V1 导联出现一个新的高大直立 T 波对缺血性心脏疾病具有 84% 的特异性（Barthwal）。

参考文献：

Barthwal SP, Agarwal R, Sarkari NB et al. Diagnostic Significance of TI < T III and TVI > TV6 signs in ischemic heart disease. J Assoc Phys India 1993；41：26 – 7

作者：**Semhar Tewelde**

心脏病

39. Statins in Acute Coronary Syndrome

1. A recent Cochrane review examined the use of early statin therapy in patients with ACS.

2. They evaluated 18 studies (14, 303 patients), which compared early statin therapy (within 14 days) to placebo or usual care.

3. The conclusion was that initiation of early statin therapy does not reduce death, myocardial infarction or stroke up to four months, but reduces the occurrence of unstable angina by 24% at 4 months following ACS.

4. Many smaller studies previously noted benefits with early statin initiation prior to this meta-analysis.

Author: Ellen Lemkin

39. 他汀类药物在急性冠状动脉 综合征(ACS)中的应用

1. 近期有一篇科可伦文献综述对 ACS 患者早期应用他汀类药物进行了评估。

2. 他们对 18 个研究报告(14, 303 个患者)在早期使用他汀类药物(14 天内)和安慰剂或常规治疗上进行了比较。

3. 结论是早期应用他汀类药物并没有减少 4 个月内死亡率、心肌梗死或脑卒中发病率,但却使 ACS 后 4 个月内的不稳定心绞痛减少了 24% 。

4. 在这个研究报告之前,有许多小型的研究报告了早期使用他汀类药物的益处。

参考文献:

Statins for acute coronary syndrome. Cochrane Database of Systemic Reviews. Volume 9, 2011.

作者: **Ellen Lemkin**

40. Monitoring dabigatran

1. Dabigatran is an oral thrombin inhibitor approved for the prevention of thromboembolism in patients with atrial fibrillation and for those undergoing orthopedic surgery.

2. In normal situations, it is not necessary to monitor any laboratory values. However, in the potential overdose situation or in the event of bleeding, it would be useful to assess the anticoagulant status.

3. The thrombin clotting time (TT) directly assesses the activity of direct thrombin inhibitors (like dabigatran), and displays a linear dose-response curve over therapeutic concentrations. At high levels, the test frequently exceeds the maximum measurements.

4. The PT and INR are less sensitive and cannot be recommended.

5. The activated partial thromboplastin time can provide qualitative assessment of anticoagulant activity but is not sensitive at supratherapeutic doses.

6. **Bottom Line**:

In emergency situations, the aPTT and TT are the most effective qualitative methods widely available for determining the presence or absence of anticoagulant effect in patients receiving dabigatran.

Author: **Ellen Lemkin**

40. 达比加群抗凝作用的监测

1.达比加群是一种预防心房颤动和骨科手术患者血栓栓塞的口服凝血酶抑制药。

2.在正常情况下，没有必要监测任何实验室指标。但是，在服药过量或有出血倾向时，监测凝血状态是有意义的。

3.凝血酶时间(TT)可用来直接反应凝血酶抑制药(如达比加群)的活性，并与剂量与治疗效果成线性关系。如剂量过高，这个结果会超过可测范围。

4.PT 和 INR 都不敏感，不建议(作为监测指标)。

5.活性部分凝血酶原时间(aPTT)可以提供量化的抗凝活性，但对于高于治疗量的剂量不敏感。

6.要点

在急诊情况下，aPTT 和 TT 是最有效的用于评价达比加群抗凝作用存在与否的定性指标。

参考文献：

Rye J, Stangier J, Haertter S, et al. Dabigatran etexilate -a novel, reversible, oral direct thrombin inhibitor: Interpretation of coagulation assays and reversal of anticoagulant activity. Thrombosis and Haemostasis 2010. 103；1116 – 1127.

作者：**Ellen Lemkin**

心脏病

41. HIV and Coronary Heart Disease (CHD)

1. HIV infected patients are at higher calculated risk for CHD compared w/ the general population of the same age.

2. HIV is known to promote atherosclerosis through mechanisms related to immune activation, chronic inflammation, coagulation disorders, and lipid disturbances.

3. Additionally combination anti-retroviral therapy (cART) has an affect on lipid and glucose metabolism demonstrated both in vitro and in vivo.

4. The presence of an accelerated process of coronary atherosclerosis in this population is a major concern.

5. Practitioners should have a high index of suspicion when confronted by young HIV patients and further data/strategies to prevent early CHD in HIV-infected patients is warranted.

Author: Semhar Tewelde

41. 艾滋病与冠状动脉心脏病

1. 与同龄人相比,艾滋病毒感染者患冠心病的风险更高。

2. 艾滋病毒通过激活免疫、慢性炎症、凝血功能障碍和血脂紊乱机制,促进动脉粥样硬化形成。

3. 此外,体内和体外试验都证实了联合抗逆转录病毒疗法(cART)对脂类和葡萄糖代谢的影响。

4. 这一人群中,冠状动脉粥样硬化进程的加快是一个相当大的问题。

5. 医护人员在治疗年轻的艾滋病患者时应该高度警惕,更多关于艾滋病患者中早期冠心病的预防的研究正在进行中。

参考文献:

Boccara F, et al. HIV and Coronary Heart Disease. J Am Coll Cardiol 2013;61:511－23

作者:Semhar Tewelde

心脏病

93

42. Secondary Prevention
in Acute Myocardial Infarction (AMI)

1. Just as aspirin is pivotal in the treatment of acute coronary syndrome, medications such as beta-blocker, statins, and angiotensin-converting enzyme inhibitors have been proven to be essential in secondary prevention of AMI.

2. Patients after AMI are typically discharged on appropriate secondary prevention medications; however the prescribed doses are often far below the proven efficacy based on clinical trials.

3. A review of 6,748 patients from 31 hospitals enrolled in 2 U. S. registries (2003 to 2008) illustrated that only 1 in 3 patients were prescribed these medications at goal doses.

4. Of patients not discharged on goal doses, up-titration during follow-up occurred infrequently ~25%.

5. Optimal medication dosing and appropriate titration is integral to prevention of further morbidity and mortality.

Author: Semhar Tewelde

42. 急性心肌梗死(AMI)的二级预防

1. 正如阿司匹林是治疗急性冠脉综合征的关键,其他药物,如 β 受体阻滞药、他汀类药物、血管紧张素转换酶抑制药,已被证明是急性心肌梗死二级预防的关键。

2. 急性心肌梗死后患者在出院时通常服用适宜的二级预防药物,但是医嘱的剂量往往远低于临床试验证明有效的量。

3. 一篇文献综述对参加美国两个登记系统(2003 年至 2008 年)31 家医院的 6 748名患者进行了总结,发现只有1/3 服用这些药物的处方剂量是符合标准的。

4. 出院时处方剂量不标准的患者,随访过程中进行再调节的大约为25%。

5. 最佳用药剂量和适当的调节是预防远期发病率和死亡率的关键。

参考文献:

Arnold S, Spertus J, Masoudi F, et al. Beyond Medication Prescription as Performace Measure:Optimal Secondary Prevention Dosing After Acute Myocardial Infarction. JACC Nov 5, 2013 Vol 62:19;1791 –1801.

作者: **Semhar Tewelde**

心
脏
病

43. Young patients and CAD

How likely is coronary artery disease to occur in young patients?

1. An autopsy series in US communities evaluated young patients (avg age 36 years old) who died of "non-natural" causes revealed coronary atherosclerosis in > 80% of the autopsy samples, with 8% having significant obstructive disease.

2. The bottom line is simple.... be wary of discounting the risk of ACS purely based on a patient's age. The HPI is the most important factor in predicting ACS.

Author: Amal Mattu

43. 年轻患者和冠心病

冠心病发生在年轻人身上的可能性有多大？

1. 一个美国尸检报告检查了非自然死亡的年轻患者（平均年龄 36 岁），发现多于 80% 的尸检样本有冠状动脉硬化，其中 8% 有严重的阻塞性疾病。

2. **要点**：要小心评价年龄在急性冠状动脉综合征发病危险因素中的作用。现病史在诊断急性冠状动脉综合征时是最重要的。

参考文献：

Nemetz PN, et al. Recent trends in the prevalance of coronary disease: a population-based autopsy study of nonnatural deaths. Arch Intern Med 2008; 168: 264 – 270.

Arbab-Zadeh A, et al. Acute coronary events. Circulation 2012; 125: 1147 – 1156.

作者：**Amal Mattu**

心
脏
病

44. Age, gender, pain, and MI outcome

1. A recent study in JAMA has provided further evidence regarding some key issues in ACS/MI presentations which seem to be commonly taught but often forgotten in actual practice.

2. Here's just a few of the key findings from this study:

1) Generally speaking, women were more likely to present without chest pain than men, and the difference between the sexes was most apparent in the <45yo groups. Overall, 42% of women presented with painless MIs. [remember from a recent prior cardiology pearl that painless MIs have a higher mortality as well]

2) Women had a higher mortality than men within the same age groups, and the difference between the sexes was most apparent in younger ages.

3) Almost 1/5 of women <45 yo with MI did not report chest pain. [We've always assumed it's just the older women that present with painless MIs... not true!]

3. A final point that should be re-stated: young women DO have MIs, they DO often present without pain, andthey DO often die. Be wary.

Author: Amal Mattu

44. 年龄、性别、疼痛和心肌梗死的预后

1. 最近在美国医学协会杂志(JAMA)发表的文章,对于我们通常了解但在实践中经常被忽略的与急性冠状动脉综合征(ACS)/心肌梗死(MI)临床表现相关的几个关键问题,提供了证据。

2. 这篇文章中涉及到的几个关键问题如下:

1)一般来讲,与男性患者相比更多的女性患者没有胸痛,差别在45岁以内最明显。42%的女性会出现无痛性心肌梗死。(记住,无痛性心肌梗死的死亡率较高。)

2)同样年纪的女性患者死亡率比男性高,越年轻差别越明显。

3)1/5的45岁以内的女性心肌梗死患者没有胸痛表现。(以前我们总认为只有老年女性才会有无痛性心肌梗死,这种想法不对!)

最后,再次重申:年轻女性也会患心肌梗死,虽然她们经常没有胸痛表现,但她们有较高的死亡率。要谨慎!

参考文献:

Canto JG, et al. Association of age and sex with myocardial infarction symptom presentation and in-hospital mortality. JAMA 2012; 307: 813 – 822.

作者: **Amal Mattu**

心脏病

45. Coronary risk factors and AMI mortality

1. We've noted studies in recent years indicating that cardiac risk factors are ineffective at predicting the likelihood of ACS in patients with acute chest pain (in other words, it's all about the HPI and EKG!).

2. Now there's evidence also that cardiac risk factors are ineffective at predicting in-hospital mortality in patients that rule in for acute MI.

3. In fact, this study actually demonstrated that in-hospital mortality is inversely related to the number of cardiac risk factors!

4. The bottom line is simple: cardiac risk factors are useful at predicting long-term risk for development of coronary artery disease, but they are NOT useful at in the acute setting.

Author: Amal Mattu

45. 冠心病危险因素与急性心肌梗死病死率

1. 最近几年我们已经了解，冠心病危险因素并不能有效地预测急性胸痛患者发生急性冠状动脉综合征的可能性(换句话说，诊断 ACS 主要依赖于现病史和心电图)。

2. 现在又有证据证实，它并不能有效地预测已明确诊断急性心肌梗死患者的住院死亡率。

3. 实际上，该研究证实住院死亡率与冠心病危险因素成反比。

4. 要点：冠心病危险因素在判断发生冠状动脉疾病长期危险方面是有用的，但在急性情况下意义不大。

参考文献：

Canto JG, Kiefe CI, Rogers WJ, et al. Number of coronary heart disease risk factors and mortality in patients with first myocardial infarction. JAMA 2011；306：2120－2127.

作者：**Amal Mattu**

心
脏
病

46. Painless MI

1. You might think that patients with painless MIs might have a better prognosis than patients with pain. Unfortunately, this is just not true.

2. As many as 1/3 of patients with proven ACS have no chest pain at presentation. Among the more common alternative presentations (anginal equivalents) are dyspnea, diaphoresis, nausea/vomiting, and syncope/near-syncope.

3. Note also that the absence of pain does not confer a better prognosis. The overall in-hospital mortality rate for patients with painless presentations is 13% vs. 4.3% for patients with chest pain.

4. A recent study supported prior literature indicating that the lack of pain is not a predictor of a more benign course, and in fact patients with painless MIs have a higher in-hospital and 1-year mortality.

5. There are several other factors that may associate lack of pain with worse outcomes (e. g. painless MIs occur more often in older patients), but regardless it's important to remember that many patients with MI will present without pain, and the lack of "typical" symptoms should not be reassuring.

Author: Amal Mattu

46. 无痛性心肌梗死

1. 你有可能认为无痛性心肌梗死的患者比有胸痛症状的患者预后好。但不幸的是，这并不正确。

2. 在被证实急性冠状综合征的患者中接近 1/3 的患者在就诊时没有胸痛症状。其他的临床表现（与心绞痛相似）包括呼吸困难，大汗，恶心/呕吐和晕厥/近晕厥。

3. 值得注意的是，没有胸痛症状并不意味着好的预后。总的住院期间死亡率在"无痛"和"有痛"患者中分别是 13% 和 4.3%。

4. 一项新的研究支持以前文献的观点，即缺乏疼痛并不意味着一个良性的过程，事实上，无痛性心肌梗死的患者住院期间和一年死亡率更高。

5. 无痛性心肌梗死的不良预后可能与很多因素有关（如无痛心肌梗死多发生在年纪大的患者），但不论怎样，一定要记住：1）很多心肌梗死的患者没有胸痛症状；2）没有典型的症状并不一定是好现象。

参考文献：

Brieger D, et al. Acute coronary syndromes without chest pain, an underdiagnosed and undertreated high-risk group: insights from the Global Registry of Acute Coronary Events. Chest 2004; 126: 461 –469.

Cho JY, et a. Comparison of outcomes of patients with painless versus painful ST-segment elevation myocardial infarction undergoing percutaneous coronary intervention. Am J Cardiol 2012; 109: 337 –343.

作者：Amal Mattu

心脏病

47. AMI in pregnancy

1. Background

1) Pregnancy is a risk factor for AMI!

(1) Acts as physiologic stress test for the heart.

(2) Increase in estrogen and progesterone.

2) Rising maternal age along with increased rates of obesity = more women w/co-morbid conditions are pregnant.

2. Incidence and types of AMI in pregnancy

1) Incidence is 6.2/100K deliveries.

2) Anterior and lateral wall MIs more common.

3. Risk factors

1) Advanced maternal age (>40yo).

2) Thrombophilia.

3) Smoking.

4) Hypertension.

5) DM.

6) Anemia & history of transfusion.

7) Complications of pregnancy.

(1) Pre-eclampsia.

(2) Post-partum hemorrhage.

(3) Post-partum infections (can induce an inflammatory state).

4. BOTTOM LINE

Young, pregnant women have MIs too!

Author: Priya Kuppusamy, MD

47.急性心肌梗死与妊娠

1.简介

1)妊娠是心肌梗死的一个危险因素!

①对心脏相当于一个负荷试验;

②雌激素和孕激素增加。

2)妊娠年龄的增加伴随肥胖率升高=更多的有慢性病的妇女怀孕。

2.妊娠期心肌梗死发病率和类型

1)发病率为6.2/10万;

2)前壁和侧壁心肌梗死比较常见。

3.危险因素

1)高龄妊娠(超过40岁);

2)高血栓形成倾向;

3)吸烟;

4)高血压;

5)糖尿病;

6)贫血和输血史;

7)妊娠合并症;

8)先兆子痫;

9)产后出血;

10)产后感染(可诱发炎症状态)。

4.要点

年轻的孕妇也可以发生心肌梗死!

参考文献:

James AH, Jamison MG, Biswas MS et al. Acute myocardial infarction in pregnancy: a United States population-based study. Circulation. 2006 Mar 28; 113(12): 1564 – 1571.

作者: **Priya Kuppusamy, MD**

心
脏
病

105

48. The HEART score for ED patients with Chest Pain

1. The diagnosis of non-STE ACS can be difficult to exclude in ED patients with chest pain. Consequently, over-diagnosis and unnecessary treatment are common. Risk stratification tools (ie. TIMI, GRACE) have been created to help risk stratify ACS patients and predict mortality. However, they are of limited utility in the ED and do not effectively differentiate low to intermediate risk patients in all-comers with chest pain.

2. The HEART score was recently prospectively validated in an ED population and was able to quickly and reliably predict risk of major adverse cardiac events (MACE-AMI, PCI, CABG, & Death).

3. 5 practical considerations (History, ECG, Age, Risk factors, & Troponin) are scored (0, 1, or 2 points each) depending on the extent of the abnormality.

1) A HEART score (0 – 10) can be quickly determined without complex calculations.

2) Low scores (0 – 3) exclude short term MACE with >98% certainty.

3) High scores (7 – 10) have high (>50%) MACE rates.

4. The HEART score performed significantly better than TIMI and GRACE scores.

5. Bottom-line: The HEART score can help to objectively risk stratify ED patients with chest pain into low, intermediate, and high risk groups. Using the HEART score can also facilitate more efficient and effective communication with colleagues.

Author: Ali Farzad

48. 急诊科胸痛患者的 HEART 评分标准

1. 非 ST 段抬高的急性冠状动脉综合征(ACS)在急诊科胸痛患者中很难排除。因此，常出现过度诊断和不必要的治疗。危险因素分析方法(如 TIMI, GRACE)可以用来帮助分析危险因素和预测死亡率。然而，它们在急诊科的应用受到限制，并不能有效区分低和中度风险的所有胸痛患者。

2. HEART 评分最近在急诊患者前瞻性研究中得到了验证，它能够快速可靠地预测主要不良心脏事件发生的风险(严重心脏不良后果 – MACE：急性心肌梗死，PCI，冠状动脉搭桥术及死亡)。

3. 对 5 个实用的因素(病史，心电图，年龄，危险因素，与肌钙蛋白)进行评分，每一项根据异常的程度给 0、1 或 2 分。

1) HEART 分数(0 ~ 10)可以不通过复杂的计算很快确定；

2) 低分数(0 ~ 3) >98% 的可能短期不会出现 MACE；

3) 高分数(7 ~ 10) MACE 发生率 >50%。

4. HEART 评分明显比 TIMI 和 GRACE 评分标准好。

5. 要点

HEART 评分标准有助于将急诊科胸痛患者的风险客观地分为低、中、高风险人群组。使用 HEART 评分标准还可以方便与同事进行更快捷、有效的沟通。

参考文献：

Backus BE, Six AJ, Kelder JC, et al. A prospective validation of the HEART score for chest pain patients at the emergency department. International Journal of Cardiology. 2013；168（3）：2153 – 2158.

http：//www. ncbi. nlm. nih. gov/pubmed/23465250

Six AJ, Backus BE, Kelder JC. Chest pain in the emergency room：value of the HEART score. Neth Heart J. 2008；16(6)：191 – 196.

http：//www. ncbi. nlm. nih. gov/pubmed/18665203

作者：**Ali Farzad**

心
脏
病

49. Coronary CT Angiography

1. CCTA vs. other tests CCTA

1) Myocardial perfusion scan & stress echo have sensitivity of 85 – 90% and specificity of 75% – 80%.

2) Negative CCTA has nearly 100% negative predicative value.

3) Radiation of CCTA 2 – 5mSv (5 – 10mSv for other nuclear medicine studies).

4) At large academic centers, cost is equal.

2. Multicenter safety study

1) Primarily looked at safety compared to other methods.

2) 5 centers, 2009 – 2011, 1370 total patients.

3) Patients age > 30, TIMI 0 – 2.

4) If CCTA negative (< 50% stenosis), < 1% had MI/death at 30 days (same as traditional group).

3. Multicenter LOS study

1) Primary outcome was LOS.

2) 9 hospitals, 2010 – 2012, total ~ 1000 patients.

3) Patients age 40 – 74.

4) CCTA had 7. 6h shorter LOS (average d/c within 8 hours of presentation to ED).

4. BOTTOM LINE

1) Only supporting evidence for CCTA is in patients with TIMI score 0 – 2.

2) Radiation from CCTA is less than other nuclear medicine studies.

3) Cost of CCTA is equal to other testing.

Author: Semhar Tewelde

美
国
急
诊
临
床
必
知
200
招

49. 冠状动脉 CT 血管造影(CCTA)

1. CCTA 与其他检查的比较

1)心肌灌注扫描和超声负荷试验的敏感性是 85% ~90%, 特异性是 75% ~80%;

2)CCTA 阴性的阴性预测值几乎接近 100%;

3)CCTA 的放射性为 2 ~5 msv(其他的同位素试验为 5 ~10);

4)在大型学术中心,收费标准一样。

2. 多中心安全研究

1)主要是与其他方法在安全方面进行比较;

2)5 个中心, 2009 - 2011 年, 1370 个患者;

3)患者年龄超过 30 岁, TIMI 分数 0 ~2;

4)如 CCTA 阴性(既小于 50% 狭窄),不到 1% 的患者 30 天内发生心肌梗死/死亡(与对照组一样)。

3. 多中心住院时间研究

1)主要指标是住院时间;

2)9 家医院, 2010 - 2012 年, 一共有大约 1000 个患者;

3)患者年龄为 40 ~74 岁;

4)CCTA 缩短了住院时间 7.6 个小时(从急诊接诊到出院平均时间为 8 小时以内)。

4. 要点

1)所有支持应用 CCTA 的证据都来源于 TIMI 分数 0 ~2 的患者(危险因素轻中度);

2)CCTA 的放射性要低于其他的同位素检查;

3)CCTA 的费用与其他检查一样。

参考文献:

Litt HI, Gatsonis C, Snyder B et al. CT angiography for safe discharge of patients with possible acute coronary syndromes. NEJM 2012; 366(15): 1393 – 403.

Hoffmann U, Truong QA, Schoenfeld DA et al. Coronary CT angiography versus standard evaluation in acute chest pain. NEJM 2012; 367(4): 299 – 308.

作者: **Semhar Tewelde**

心脏病

50. Cardiogenic shock

1. CS is most commonly secondary to a large MI where >40% of the myocardium is involved; however mechanical, valvular, dysrhythmogenic, and infectious etiologies should also be considered: papillary or chordal dysfunction, free wall or septal defects disease, insuffiency of any valve, myopericarditis, endocarditis, Takotsubo, end stage cardiomyopathy, and tamponade.

2. Incidence of 5% – 10% STEMI and 2.5 – 5% NSTEMI

3. Mortality ~ 50%

4. Immediate coronary reperfusion is the best treatment (NNT 8). Medical therapy is a distant second choice in management, with reperfusion and pressors as needed. Early intra-aortic balloon pump use is key.

5. Recent case reports have shown imporved outcomes when induced hypothermia was used in patients refractory to traditional therapy with pressors/inotropes/IABP.

6. There are only a few interventions that have been demonstrated to improve outcomes: early use of intra-aortic balloon pump, stenting, and G2B3A inhibitors.

7. It is generally recommended to avoid clopidogrel since so many of these patients will require CABG.

8. Early use of mechanical ventilation decreases work of breathing and improves oxygenation.

9. Remember that age alone is not a contraindication to aggressive treatment.

Author: Amal Mattu

50. 心源性休克

1. 心源性休克最常见于大面积(超过40%)的心肌梗死;但同时还要考虑机械性、瓣膜、心律失常和感染性原因:乳头肌和索功能失调、心脏房室壁或房间隔缺陷、任何瓣膜功能异常、心肌心包炎、心内膜炎、压力诱导(Takotsubo)心肌病、晚期心肌病和心包填塞。

2. 发病率占ST段抬高型心肌梗死患者的5%~10%和非ST段抬高型心肌梗死的2.5%~5%。

3. 死亡率约50%。

4. 紧急冠状动脉再通是首选的治疗手段(需要治疗的病例数-NNT为8)。包括溶栓和升压药在内的药物治疗方案都是次选。早期应用主动球囊反搏是相当关键的。

5. 最近有病例报告显示,对包括升压药/强心药/主动脉球囊反搏等传统治疗方法无效的患者,低温治疗会改善预后。

6. 只有几种治疗方法能够改善预后:早期主动脉球囊反搏、支架和G2B3A抑制药。

7. 通常建议不要使用氯吡格雷,因为很多这样的患者都需要冠状动脉搭桥术。

8. 早期使用机械通气有助于减轻呼吸负荷和改善氧供。

9. 要记住,年龄并不是积极治疗的禁忌证。

作者:Amal Mattu

51. To Pump or not to Pump?

1. Intra-aortic balloon pumps (IABP) are devices that provide hemodynamic support during cardiogenic shock; the balloon inflates during diastole (improving coronary artery perfusion) and deflates during systole (reducing afterload and improving systemic perfusion).

2. Several guidelines recommend placement of an IABP for patients in cardiogenic shock secondary to acute myocardial infarction (AMI), if early revascularization (e. g., CABG) is planned (Class I recommendation). Data behind this recommendation, however, is limited.

3. The IABP-SHOCK II trial was a randomized, multi-center, open-label study that enrolled 600 patients (598 in the analysis) with cardiogenic shock secondary to AMI (STEMI or NSTEMI). Patients were randomized to the control group (receiving standard therapy; N = 298) or the experimental group (receiving IABP; N = 300).

4. No significant difference was found between groups with respect to 30 – day mortality (primary end-point), secondary end-points (e. g., time to hemodynamic stabilization, renal function, lactate levels, etc.), or complications (e. g., major bleeding, peripheral ischemic complications, etc.).

5. Bottom line: Perhaps it is time to reassess the approach to cardiogenic shock secondary to AMI when early revascularization is planned. At this time consultation with local expertise is recommended.

Author: Haney Mallemat

51. 是用泵还是不用泵?

1. 主动脉球囊反搏(IABP)是在心源性休克治疗中用来提供血流动力学支持的设备。球囊在舒张期充气(改善冠状动脉灌注),收缩期放气(减轻后负荷,以改善全身灌注)。

2. 多个临床指南都建议在急性心肌梗死造成的心源性休克时使用 IABP,以过渡到早期血管再通治疗(如冠状动脉搭桥等,一级建议)。但是,支持这一建议的数据有限。

3. 主动脉球囊反搏 - 休克(IABP-SHOCK)II 研究是一项随机的,多中心的,开放标签的临床研究,包括了 600 个(598 个用于分析)由急性心肌梗死(ST 段抬高或不抬高)造成心源性休克的患者。患者随机的分成对照组(接受标准治疗,298 人)或实验组(接受 IABP,300 人)。

4. 结果显示在 30 天死亡率(主要指标)、血流动力学稳定时间,肾功能,乳酸水平(次要指标)或合并症(大出血,外周缺血)方面两组之间没有明显差别。

5. 要点

对于有计划要接受早期再灌注治疗的急性心肌梗死心源性休克的患者,其抢救方案要进行重新评估。目前,专家意见正在收集中。

参考文献:

Thiele, H. et al. Intra aortic balloon support for myocardial infarction with cardiogenic shock. NEJM 2012 Oct 4; 367(14): 1287 – 1296.

作者: **Haney Mallemat**

心
脏
病

52. Cardiogenic shock and clopidogrel

1. Patients with ACS are often treated early with clopidogrel. However, if the patient with ACS appears to be developing cardiogenic shock, its probably best to withhold the early clopidogrel.

2. The literature indicates that patients with cardiogentic shock benefit most from emergent PCI, and many of these patients will need CABG. Generally it's best to avoid clopidogrel in patients heading for CABG.

3. The use of clopidogrel in patients with cardiogenic shock can be deferred to the cardiologists in the cath lab once they decide whether the patient will need CABG or not.

Author: Amal Mattu

52. 心源性休克与氯吡格雷

1. 急性冠状动脉综合征(ACS)的患者通常应尽快给予氯吡格雷。但是,如果患者有发生心源性休克的迹象,最好不要用。

2. 目前文献显示:对发生心源性休克的患者最有效的治疗方法是紧急经皮冠状动脉介入治疗(percutaneous coronary intervention, PCI),其中很多患者可能需要冠状动脉搭桥术(coronary artery bypass graft, CABG)。一般来说,最好避免对这些有可能需要 CABG 的患者使用氯吡格雷。(此药可增加 CABG 患者的出血倾向。)

3. 对心源性休克的患者是否使用氯吡格雷,可由导管室的心脏科医生根据患者是否需要 CABG 来决定。

参考文献:

Thiele H, Allam B, Chatellier G, et al. Shock in acute myocardial infarction: the Cape Horn for trials? Eur Heart J 2010; 31: 1828 – 1835.

作者: **Amal Mattu**

心脏病

53. B-Type Natriuretic Peptide

1. B-type natriuretic peptide (BNP) is a useful prognostic biomarker in patients with reduced LVEF, but data in heart failure (HF) with preserved ejection fraction (HFPEF) is minimal.

2. A recent study sought to determine the prognostic value of BNP in patients with HFPEF in comparison to data in HF patients with reduced left ventricular EF <40%.

3. 615 patients with mild to moderate HF were followed for 18 months and BNP was measured at baseline and related to the primary outcomes (mortality and HF hospitalization).

4. BNP levels were significantly higher in patients with reduced LVEF than in those with HFPEF ($p < 0.001$), however the risk of adverse outcomes and prognosis in patients with HFPEF is as poor as in those with reduced LVEF.

Author: Semhar Tewelde

53. B 型利钠肽

1. B 型利钠肽(BNP)对左室功能减低的心力衰竭患者是一个可靠的判断预后的生物指标,但在左室射血分数正常的心力衰竭(HFPEF)患者中的数据却非常有限。

2. 最近的一项研究评估了 BNP 对 HFPEF 患者的预后价值,并与左室 EF < 40% 的心力衰竭患者进行了比较。

3. 615 例轻度至中度心力衰竭患者在测量了 BNP 水平后随访了 18 个月,观察了 BNP 与主要指标 (死亡率和心力衰竭住院率)的关系。

4. 左室 EF 降低患者的 BNP 水平明显高于那些 HFPEF 患者($P < 0.001$),但是 HFPEF 患者的预后和那些左室 EF 降低的患者一样不佳。

参考文献：

B-Type Natriuretic Peptide and Prognosis in Heart Failure Patients With Preserved and Reduced Ejection Fraction. Veldhuisen D, Linssen G, et al. J Am Coll Cardiol 2013; 61: 1498 – 506

作者: **Semhar Tewelde**

心
脏
病

54. Atrial Fibrillation

1. Atrial fibrillation is most commonly associated with cardiovascular disease.

2. Non cardiac causes: pulmonary disease/PE, hyperthyroidism, sympathomimetics, drugs/ETOH.

3. AFFIRM & RACE trials compared outcomes of a fib patients treated w/ rate vs. rhythm control.

4. No significant difference in survival between groups.

5. Risk of thromboembolic CVA.

Rhythm control = Rate control + anticoagulation

6. New data challenges the need for strict heart rate control.

7. Resting heart rate should be < 110 bpm.

8. Use CHADS2 score to identify who requires anticoagulation based on % risk of emboli.

Chronic heart failure, HTN, Age > 75, DM, Stroke/TIA.

Author: Semhar Tewelde

54. 心房颤动

1. 心房颤动主要与心血管疾病有关。

2. 非心脏原因: 肺部疾病/肺动脉栓塞, 甲状腺功能亢进, 交感神经兴奋, 药物/酒精。

3. AFFIRM/RACE 临床研究对心房颤动患者控制心率和控制心律治疗后的预后进行了比较。

4. 两组患者的生存率没有显著差异。

5. 血栓或栓塞性脑血管意外(CVA)危险性

控制心律 = 控制心率 + 抗凝治疗。

6. 新的数据对严格心率控制提出了质疑。

7. 静息状态下心率低于 110 次/分即可。

8. 应用 CHADS2 评分标准来确定血栓形成的危险度, 以决定是否接受(长期)抗凝治疗。

慢性心力衰竭(CHF), 高血压(HTN), 年龄超过 75 岁, 糖尿病, 脑卒中/短暂性脑缺血(TIA)。

参考文献:

Atrial Fibrillation. Bontempo L, Goralnick E. Emerg Med Clin N Am 29 (2011) 747 – 758.

作者: **Semhar Tewelde**

心
脏
病

55. Risk factors for atrial fibrillation

1. A proper understanding of the risk factors associated with atrial fibrillation (AF) development may potentially decrease the risk of AF.

2. Metabolic syndrome-Patients with metabolic syndrome have demonstrated a higher risk of AF.

3. Obstructive sleep apnea-Patients with severe obstructive sleep apnea (OSA) and AF may have a decreased response to antiarrhythmic drug therapy compared with patients with no OSA or less severe OSA and may be at a higher risk for AF ablation failure.

4. Alcohol-The relationship between alcohol use and the development of AF is dose dependent, with higher amounts of alcohol associated with increased risk of AF and probably some increase in AF even at low doses of alcohol.

5. Exercise-Extreme exercise has been linked to potential cardiotoxicity, including an increased risk of AF.

6. Vitmin D- Excessive vitamin D intake (>100ng/ml) may be associated with an increased risk of AF.

7. Omega – 3 polyunsaturated fatty acids- The role of omega – 3 polyunsaturated fatty acids in setting of AF is controversial. Although some studies demonstrate a lower incidence of AF recurrence with omega – 3 polyunsaturated fatty acids use, others have shown an increased risk.

8. Coffee and tea- Drinking moderate coffee and tea does not cause AF and may even decrease its occurrence.

Author: Feng Xiao

55.对心房颤动危险因素的新认识

1.正确理解与心房颤动(AF)的发展相关的危险因素会减少心房颤动的风险。

2.代谢综合征——代谢综合征患者已被证明有很高的 AF 风险。

3.阻塞性睡眠呼吸暂停(OSA)——与无 OSA 或不太严重的 OSA 相比,重度 OSA 伴 AF 患者对抗心律失常药物治疗的反应性下降并更可能使心房颤动消融治疗失败。

4.酒精——酒精和 AF 之间的关系与剂量有关,较高量的酒精可增加 AF 的危险,即使低剂量的酒精也可能会增加 AF 的风险。

5.锻炼——过量运动已被证实具有潜在的心脏毒性,包括增加 AF 风险。

6.维生素 D——过量的维生素 D 摄入(>100 ng/mL),可增加 AF 风险。

7.Omega - 3 多不饱和脂肪酸——Omega - 3 多不饱和脂肪酸对 AF 的作用是有争议的。一些研究表明:Omega - 3 多不饱和脂肪酸的使用可降低 AF 危险,但另一些文献却报告它增加了 AF 风险。

8.咖啡和茶——饮用适量的咖啡和茶,不会造成 AF,甚至可能降低其发生。

参考文献:

Mayo Clin Proc 2013;88(4):394 - 409.

作者:肖锋（Feng Xiao）

心脏病

56. Reversal of warfarin in 2012

1. INR can be influenced by a number of factors

1) 400 drug-drug interactions with warfarin.

2) Food.

3) Alcohol.

4) Disease states.

2. major categories for patients with elevated INR

1) No bleeding or minor bleeding.

2) Major bleeding.

3. No bleeding and mildly elevated INR (INR of 3 – 5)

1) Spontaneous events are uncommon.

2) Relative risk is 2.7 of spontaneous bleeding events.

3) Most patients can just have their warfarin held for a day or two.

4) Consider treatment in patient with some risky disease states.

(1) Advanced age.

(2) Active malignancy.

(3) CHF.

5) Can give IV or oral vitamin K 2.5 mg

4. No bleeding and significantly elevated INR (INR >5)

1) Relative risk of spontaneous bleeding goes up to 21.8.

2) Give IV or oral vitamin K 2.5 – 5mg.

3) Should not give subcutaneous vitamin K ever.

5. Minor bleeding and elevated INR

1) Hold warfarin.

2) Give IV or oral vitamin K 5 mg.

6. Major bleeding and elevated INR

1) Vitamin K IV 10 mg slowly.

2) Minor risk of anaphylaxis (3 out of 10,000 patients).

3) Fresh frozen plasma or FFP

(1) 10 – 15 mL/kg dosing.

(2) Takes a little time to work and to get ready.

(3) Readily available in most hospitals.

4) Prothrombin complex concentrate or PCC

(1) Has more vitamin K clotting factors.

(2) Version available in the US only has 3 factors and very little factor VII.

(3) Usually has to be given in combination with factor VII.

(4) Has a 1.8% risk of arterial thrombosis.

5) Recombinant activated factor VII

(1) Short half-life of 2 - 6 hours.

(2) Higher risk of arterial thrombosis, 10%.

Author: Ellen Lemkin

心
脏
病

56.2012 年纠正华法林过量的指南

1.INR 可被很多因素影响

1）有 400 种药物与华法林有相互反应；

2）食物；

3）酒精；

4）疾病状态。

2.INR 增高的患者可分两类

1）没有或有轻微出血；

2）大出血。

3.没有出血，INR 轻度增高（3~5）

1）自发性出血不常见；

2）自发性出血的相对危险度是 2.7；

3）许多患者只要停药 1~2 天即可；

4）有下列几种危险疾病状态的要考虑治疗。

(1)年纪很大；

(2)活动期的恶性肿瘤；

(3)心力衰竭。

5）可以静脉或口服维生素 K 2.5 mg，

4.没有出血，INR 明显增高（超过 5）

1）自发性出血的相对危险度增至 21.8；

2）可以静脉或口服维生素 K 5 mg；

3）任何时候都不要皮内注射维生素 K。

5.轻度出血，INR 升高

1）停用华法林；

2）静脉或口服维生素 K 5 mg。

6.大出血，INR 升高

1）缓慢静脉注射维生素 K 10 mg；

2）过敏反应风险很小（发生率约为 3/10000）；

3）新鲜冰冻血浆（FFP）

(1)剂量：10~15 mL/kg；

（2）不需要太长的时间准备；

（3）很多医院都有。

4）凝血酶原复合物浓缩剂（PCC）

（1）含更多的维生素 K 依赖性凝血因子；

（2）美国市场的 PCC 主要含 3 个因子和非常少的凝血因子Ⅶ；

（3）一般与凝血因子Ⅶ同时用；

（4）动脉血栓的危险为 1.8%。

5）生物合成的凝血因子Ⅶ

（1）半衰期为 2～6 小时；

（2）较高的动脉血栓形成危险，发生率约为 10%。

参考文献：

Garcia DA，Crowther MA. Reversal of warfarin，case-based practice recommendations. Circulation. 2012；125：2944 – 2947.

作者：**Ellen Lemkin**

心
脏
病

57. Life-Threatening Causes of Syncope

1. Syncope is a sudden lack of blood supply to the brain typically caused by a problem in the regulation of blood pressure or a problem with the heart.

2. Syncope can be broadly classified in 3 categories neural reflex (~60%), orthostatic (~15%), and cardiac (~15%).

3. Even in the absence of a firm diagnosis of cardiac syncope, the presence of known structural heart disease (CAD) or evidence a primary electrical disorder is associated with a poor prognosis.

4. Cardiac causes of syncope can also be divided into 3 categories: structural heart disease, obstructive lesions, and arrhythmogenic potential.

1) Structural: Ischemic heart disease, dilated cardiomyopathy, etc.

2) Obstructive: HCM, aortic/mitral stenosis, atrial myxoma, pulmonary HTN, PE, tamponade.

3) Arrhythmogenic:

(1) Brady: AV block, sick sinus, sinus arrest/pause.

(2) Tachy: SVT (AVNRT/AVRT), accessory pathways (WPW), or primary arrhythmias.

Author: Semhar Tewelde

美
国
急
诊
临
床
必
知
200
招

57. 危及生命的晕厥

1.晕厥是由突发的大脑血液供应不足所致,通常由血压调节紊乱或心脏问题引起。

2.晕厥大致可分为3类:神经反射性(60%)、体位性(15%)和心源性(15%)。

3.即使在没有明确心源性晕厥诊断的情况下,已知的结构性心脏疾病(CAD)或电传导紊乱都与不良预后相关。

4.心源性晕厥的原因也可分为3类:器质性心脏疾病、阻塞性病变和潜在的心律失常。

1)结构性:缺血性心脏疾病、扩张型心肌病等。

2)阻塞性:肥厚性心肌病、主动脉瓣/二尖瓣狭窄、心房黏液瘤、肺高压、肺栓塞,心包填塞。

3)心律失常因素

(1)过缓:病态窦房结综合征、房室传导阻滞、窦性停搏/静止

(2)过速:室上性心动过速(房室结折返性心动过速/房室折返性心动过速)、旁路(WPW)或原发性心律失常

作者: **Semhar Tewelde**

58. Brugada Syndrome

1. Autosomal dominant inherited arrhythmic disorder characterized by mutation in sodium-channels.

2. Arrhythmic events are often observed at rest or while asleep, resulting in VF and SCD.

3. Diagnostic criteria consists of 2 parts: (1) ECG abnormalities (2) clinical characteristics.

4. ECG abnormalities: incomplete or complete RBBB in right precordial leads (V1 – V2).

1) Type Ⅰ: coved-type ST segment elevation and negative T wave.

2) Type Ⅱ: saddle-back ST segment elevation followed by a positive or biphasic T wave.

3) Type Ⅲ: ST segment elevation without meeting criteria for type Ⅰ or Ⅱ variants.

5. Clinical characteristics: hx of VT/VF, family hx of SCD or abnormal ECG, agonal respirations during sleep, or inducible VT/VF during EP study.

Author: Semhar Tewelde

58. Brugada 综合征

1.常染色体显性遗传的心律失常,由钠离子通道基因突变造成。

2.心律失常经常在休息或睡眠时发生,表现为心室颤动和心脏性猝死。

3.诊断标准包括心电图异常和临床表现特征。

4.心电图异常:右胸前导联(V1 – V2)不完全或完全性右束支传导阻滞。

1)Ⅰ型:ST 段拱形抬高和倒置 T 波;

2)Ⅱ型:ST 段鞍背形抬高和正向或双向 T 波;

3)Ⅲ型:ST 段抬高但又不符合如上Ⅰ和Ⅱ型的标准。

5.临床特点:室性心动过速或心室颤动的病史,心脏性猝死或异常心电图家族史,睡眠时有呼吸暂停或在心脏电生理检查时可诱发室性心动过速/心室颤动。

参考文献:

Mizusawa Y, Wilde A. Brugada Syndrome. Circ Arrhythm Electrophysiol. 2012;5:606 – 616.

作者:Semhar Tewelde

心脏病

59. Bi & Tri-fascicular Blocks

1. Bifascicular block

1) Right bundle branch block (RBBB) + left anterior fascicular block (LAFB).

2) RBBB + left posterior fascicular block (LPFB).

2. Incomplete Trifascicular block

1) Bifascicular block w/1st degree AV block, classically referred to as "trifascicular block".

2) Bifascicular block w/2nd degree AV block.

3) Alternating LBBB + RBBB.

3. Complete Trifascicular block

Bifascicular block w/3rd degree AV block.

Author: Semhar Tewelde

59. 双束支和三束支传导阻滞

1. 双束支传导阻滞

1）右束支传导阻滞（RBBB）+左前分支阻滞（LAFB）；

2）右束支传导阻滞（RBBB）+左后分支阻滞（LPFB）。

2. 不完全性三束传导支阻滞

1）双束支传导阻滞伴 1 度房室传导阻滞，这是经典的"三束支传导阻滞"；

2）双束支阻滞伴 2 度房室传导阻滞；

3）左束支传导阻滞和右束支传导阻滞交替出现。

3. 完全三束支传导阻滞

双束支传导阻滞伴 3 度房室传导阻滞。

参考文献：

Surawicz B, Knilans T. Chou's Electrocardiography in Clinical Practice（6th edition），Saunders 2008.

Wagner, GS. Marriott's Practical Electrocardiography（11th edition），Lippincott Williams & Wilkins 2007.

Levis J, Garmel G. Clinical Emergency Medicine Casebook, Cambridge University Press 2009.

作者：**Semhar Tewelde**

心
脏
病

60. Prosthetic Heart Valves

1. 90,000 artificial heart valves are implanted yearly in USA/ 280,000 yearly worldwide.

2. Mechanical Valves (synthetic material)

1) Caged Ball.

2) Monoleaflet (tilting disc).

3) Bileaflet.

4) High risk of thromboembolism.

5) Requires lifelong anticoagulation.

6) Good long term durability.

3. Bioprosthetic/Xenograft Valves (biological tissue)

1) Porcine.

2) Bovine.

3) Low risk of thromboembolism.

4) No long term anticoagulation.

5) Poor long term durability (especially in young and pregnant populations).

4. Complications

1) Primary valve failure.

2) Endocarditis.

3) Thrombus/Embolus.

4) Mechanical hemolytic anemia.

5) Anticoagulation related hemorrhage.

6) Myocardial abscess.

New atrioventricular (AV) block + artificial valve = myocardial abscess (until proven otherwise).

Author: Semhar Tewelde

60. 人工心脏瓣膜

1. 美国每年有 9 万例人工心脏瓣膜的置入，全世界有 28 万例。

2. 机械瓣膜(合成材料)

1) 笼罩球瓣；

2) 单瓣膜(倾斜盘)；

3) 双瓣膜；

4) 血栓形成和栓塞的危险度高；

5) 需要终身的抗凝治疗；

6) 瓣膜寿命长。

3. 生物/异体瓣膜(生物组织)

1) 猪；

2) 牛；

3) 血栓形成和栓塞的危险度低；

4) 不需要长期抗凝治疗；

5) 瓣膜寿命短(尤其对于年轻和怀孕的患者)。

4. 合并症

1) 瓣膜功能衰竭；

2) 心内膜炎；

3) 血栓/栓塞；

4) 机械性溶血性贫血；

5) 与抗凝治疗有关的出血；

6) 心肌脓肿。

新发生的房室传导阻滞 + 人工瓣膜 = 心肌脓肿(除非证实有其他原因)。

参考文献：

Pibarot P, Dumesnil J. Prosthetic Heart Valves: Selection of the Optimal Prosthesis and Long-Term Management. Circulation. Vol 119(7); 24 Feb 2009, pp 1034 – 1048.

作者：**Semhar Tewelde**

心脏病

133

61. Cardiac Screening in Young Athletes

1. Sports are associated w/an increased risk for sudden cardiac death (SCD) in athletes who are affected by cardiovascular conditions predisposing to ventricular arrhythmias (VA).

2. SCD has substantially decreased in Veneto Italy due to the introduction of a preparticipation screening program that identifies unrecognized cardiovascular conditions.

3. This study included 145 athletes evaluated for VA using a screening protocol of ECG, exercise testing, echocardiography, holter monitoring, and cardiac MRI.

4. ECG was normal in most athletes (>85%).

5. VA were detected prevalently during exercise testing.

6. Cardiac MRI detected right ventricular regional kinetic abnormalities (ARVD) in 9 of 30 athletes.

7. A total of 30% of these athletes had potentially dangerous VA.

8. In asymptomatic athletes w/prevalently normal ECG, most VA's can be identified by adding an exercise test.

Author: Semhar Tewelde

61. 年轻运动员的心脏检查

1. 运动对于有可以导致室性心律失常心血管疾病的运动员来说，将增加发生心脏性猝死（SCD）的危险。

2. SCD 在意大利威尼托已明显下降，主要原因是实施了一个在参加运动前能够发现还没有诊断的心脏病的项目。

3. 这一研究包括了 145 个运动员，通过 ECG、运动试验、超声心动图、动态心电监测和心脏核磁共振来评价产生室性心律失常的可能性。

4. 多数运动员的心电图都正常（超过 85%）。

5. 室性心律失常主要发生在运动试验期间。

6. 心脏磁共振在 30 名运动员中发现了 9 名有局部右室壁活动异常。

7. 在这些运动员中，30% 有潜在的发生室性心律失常的危险。

8. 对于心电图正常又无症状的运动员，多数室性心律失常可以通过运动试验来诊断。

参考文献：

Steriotis A，Nava A，et al. Noninvasive Cardiac Screening in Young Athletes With Ventricular Arrhythmias. The American Journal of Cardiology. Feb 2013：111；4，557 – 562.

作者：**Semhar Tewelde**

心脏病

62. Infections of Implanted Cardiac Devices

1. Risk factors

1) Highest with AICDs (regardless of lead placement site) −2% infection rate at 5 years.

2) Renal failure.

3) Complications at generator incision site.

4) Devices with multiple leads.

5) Re-implantations actually associated with fewer infections.

2. Infection characteristics

1) Most infections d/t S. aureus (rapid onset) and coagulase-negative staph (indolent).

2) 30% of infections do not occur at generator site (lead infection or endocarditis).

3. Management

1) Don't aspirate seromas or hematomas (should be done in OR).

2) Get blood cultures (35% positive in cases of proven infection) BEFORE antibiotics.

3) If concern for endocarditis, go straight to TEE.

4) Definitive treatment is to remove everything and treat with antibiotics for 4 − 6 weeks.

4. BOTTOM LINE

Consider endocarditis in patients with implanted cardiac devices and fever/constitutional symptoms.

Author: Michael Bond, MD

62. 植入式心脏装置的感染

1.危险因素

1)感染率最高的是自动植入式心律转复除颤器(与导线的位置无关)——5年内的感染率为2%;

2)肾功能衰竭;

3)在电源器切口部位发生并发症;

4)多导联装置;

5)重新植入实际上减少了感染。

2.感染特点

1)大多数感染是由于金黄色葡萄球菌(快速发作)和凝固酶阴性葡萄球菌(缓发型);

2)30%的感染不发生在电源器部位(导线感染或感染性心内膜炎)。

3.处理

1)不要抽吸黏液肿或血肿(应在手术室进行);

2)在使用抗生素前做血培养(在证实的感染病例中阳性率为35%);

3)如果怀疑心内膜炎,直接做经食道超声心动图;

4)根治性的治疗方法是清除感染源,并用抗生素治疗4~6周。

4.要点

对有发热/全身症状的有植入性心脏设备的患者要考虑感染性心内膜炎。

参考文献:

Baddour LM, Cha YM, Wilson WR. Infections of cardiovascular implantable electronic devices. N Eng Med 2012, 367(9): 842 – 849.

Poole JE, Gleva MJ, Mela T et al. Complication rates associated with pacemaker or implantable cardioverter-defibrillator generator replacements and upgrade procedures: results from the REPLACE registry. Circulation, 2010, 122(16): 1553 – 1561.

作者: **Michael Bond, MD**

心脏病

63. Postural Tachycardia Syndrome

1. Postural tachycardia syndrome (POTS) is defined as orthostatic intolerance w/ an increase in heart rate by 30 bpm (or HR > 120 bpm) that occurs within 10 mins of standing or upright tilt.

2. Orthostatic intolerance due to POTS will NOT cause orthostatic hypotension (defined as fall of > 20/10 mm Hg on standing); instead patients may display no change, a small decline, or even a modest increase in blood pressure.

3. Symptoms include: palpitations, fatigue, lightheadedness, exercise intolerance, nausea, diminished concentration, tremulousness, and syncope.

4. POTS is a heterogeneous group of disorders with similar clinical manifestations

1) Primary POTS – partial dysautonomia form.

2) Secondary POTS – hyperadrenergic form.

5. Tx varies according to the subtype/etiology of POTS and must be individualized.

6. Caveat: inappropriate sinus tachycardia (IST) and POTS are two different diagnosis where significant overlap exists, however the tachycardia in IST is NOT postural.

Author: Semhar Tewelde

63. 体位性心动过速综合征

1. 体位性心动过速综合征(POTS)被定义为直立不耐受伴，在卧位转为站立或倾斜 10 分钟内，心率增加 30 次/min(或 HR >120 次/min)。

2. 由 POTS 所造成的体位不耐受将不引起体位性低血压(定义为站立时血压下降 >20/10 mmHg)，患者的血压反而可能会表现为没有变化；一个小的下降，甚至可能会升高。

3. 症状：心悸、乏力、头晕、运动耐受力下降、恶心、注意力不集中、震颤和晕厥。

4. POTS 是一组有相似临床表现的不同性质疾病群

1)原发性 POTS——部分自主神经功能障碍所致；

2)继发 POTS——高肾上腺素所致。

5. 治疗根据 POTS 的不同亚型/病因，必须个体化。

6. 注意：不典型的窦性心动过速(IST)和 POTS 是两个不同的诊断，存在明显的重叠，但是 IST 的心动过速并不因体位而变化。

参考文献：

Grubb B. Postural Tachycardia Syndrome. Circulation, 2008, 117: 2814 – 2817.

作者：**Semhar Tewelde**

心
脏
病

64. Dextrocardia

1. Mirror-image dextrocardia is the most common form of cardiac malposition and is commonly associated with situsinversus of the abdominal organs.

2. The anatomic right ventricle is anterior to the left ventricle and the aortic arch curves to the right and posteriorly.

3. 25% percent of these patients will have associated sinusitis and bronchiectasis (Kartagener's syndrome).

4. ECG changes associated with dextrocardia include:

1) Right-axis deviation.

2) Global negativity in leads I and aVL (negative QRS w/inverted P and T waves).

3) Lead aVR similar to the normal aVL (positive QRS).

4) Absent R wave progression in precordial leads/dominant S waves.

Author: SemharTewelde

64. 右位心

1. 镜像关系的右位心是心脏异位的最常见形式，常伴有腹腔脏器转位。
2. 解剖上，右心室位于左心室前方；主动脉弓向右后方向弯曲。
3. 25％的患者伴有鼻窦炎和支气管扩张（Kartagener 氏综合征）。
4. 与右位心有关的心电图改变包括：

1）电轴右偏；
2）I 和 aVL 导联全部负波（负性 QRS 伴 P 和 T 波倒置）；
3）aVR 导联与正常 aVL 类似（正 QRS）；
4）胸前导联无 R 波逐渐增高/明显的 S 波。

参考文献：

Al-Khadra A. Mirror-Image Dextrocardia With SitusInversus. Circulation, 1995, 91: 1602 –1603.

作者：SemharTewelde

心脏病

65. Novel Therapy in Ascending Aortic Dissection

1. Stanford type A (proximal) aortic dissection accounts for ~60% of all aortic dissections.

2. Classic treatment includes direct surgical replacement of the ascending aorta w/ prosthetic graft (+/ - aortic valve repair/replacement).

3. 20% - 30% of these patients (institutional dependent) are considered poor candidates for surgery and receive only medical management, which innately results in substandard outcomes.

4. In this study those who were considered poor candidates for surgical repair underwent novel endovascular treatment.

5. Endovascular repair in this study was considered both appropriate and improved traditional medical outcomes in patients who were considered poor candidates.

Author: Semhar Tewelde

美国急诊临床必知200招

65. 升主动脉夹层的新疗法

1. Stanford A 型(近端)约占所有主动脉夹层的60%。

2. 经典的治疗包括直视下升主动脉人工血管置换术(+/- 主动脉瓣修补或置换)。

3. 这些患者中的20%~30%(因医疗机构而异)被认为不适合做手术，只能保守治疗，最终导致不良后果。

4. 在这项研究中，对那些被认为不适合做手术的患者进行了新型的血管内治疗。

5. 在这项研究中的血管内修补对不适合做手术患者是可行的并能改善传统的治疗效果。

参考文献：

Lu Q，Feng J，et al. Endovascular Repair of Ascending Aortic Dissection A Novel Treatment Option for Patients Judged Unfit for Direct Surgical Repair. J Am Coll Cardiol, 2013, 61: 1917 – 1924.

作者：**Semhar Tewelde**

心脏病

66. Takayasu Arteritis（TA）

1. Takayasu arteritis（TA）is a granulomatous vasculitis that affects the aorta and its major branches.

2. Involvement of the aortic arch is associated w/CNS symptoms, claudication, absent peripheral pulses, and cardiac manifestations.

3. The EULAR/PReS consensus criteria for Dx of childhood TA requires characteristic angiographic abnormalities of the aorta plus 1 of the following:

1）Absent peripheral pulses or claudication.

2）Blood pressure discrepancy in any limb.

3）Bruits.

4）Hypertension.

5）Elevated acute phase reactants.

4. Gold standard for Dx is angiography; however, CT and MR angiograms are less invasive and can detect inflammation & luminal diameter changes.

5. Tx is challenging, steroids may induce remission in up to 60% p.

Author: Semhar Tewelde

66. 多发性大动脉炎

1. 多发性大动脉炎(TA)是累及主动脉及其大分支的肉芽肿性血管炎。

2. 主动脉弓的病变会引起中枢神经系统症状、间歇性跛行、末梢动脉搏动消失和心脏方面的表现。

3. 欧洲抗风湿病联盟(EULAR)/欧洲儿童风湿病学会(PRES)共同标准,诊断儿童多发性大动脉炎需要特异性的主动脉造影异常,同时包括下列一项:

1) 末梢动脉搏动丧失或间歇性跛行;

2) 任何肢体间的血压差异;

3) 血管杂音;

4) 高血压;

5) 急性期反应产物增加。

4. 确诊的金标准是动脉造影,但 CTA 和 MRA 不仅创伤性低,还可以发现炎症和腔内径的改变。

5. 治疗是具有挑战性的,激素可能对大约60%的患者有效。

参考文献:

Weiss P, et al. Pediatric vasculitis. The Pediatric clinics of North America. April, 2012, 59(2): 407 - 423.

作者: Semhar Tewelde

心脏病

危重病
Critical Care Medicine

67. Critical care studies in the last 5 years that change our practice

1. Fluid management in ARDS

1) Patients did better with conservative ("dry") fluid management at day 7.

2) No difference in mortality, but there was a difference in:

(1) Oxygenation.

(2) Plateau pressures.

(3) Time on ventilator.

(4) Time in ICU.

3) PA catheter vs CVP.

4) In the ED, still should fluid resuscitate, but once hypotension & markers of end-organ dysfunction improve, back off on fluid (goal is equal I&Os, CVP = 4).

2. Glucose control (permissive mild hyperglycemia)

1) Intensive control (81 - 108) has higher incidence of severe hypoglycemia and worsened outcomes compared to conventional control (< 180).

2) Too much sugar is bad (> 200), but too little sugar is REALLY bad.

3) Use insulin drip instead of bolus dose.

3. Corticosteroids in septic shock

1) Clear that high dose steroids worsen outcomes.

2) Low dose steroids result in shorter duration of shock, but no overall improvement in 28 - day mortality, and higher incidence of secondary infections.

3) Should not be give to all comers.

4) Still recommended for patients who have refractory septic shock, not responding to IVF or vasopressors (50mg hydrocortisone IV bolus followed by continuous infusion at 200 mg/24 h).

5) Should see response within 1 - 2 hours.

4. Vasopressor therapy in shock

1) As second (add-on) vasopressors, no difference in mortality between vasopressin & norepinephrine.

2) Dopamine compared to norepinephrine as first line agents.

3) No significant difference in mortality at 28 days.

4) Higher incidence of arrhythmias in dopamine patients.

5) Increased mortality in subgroup of patients with cardiogenic shock who got dopamine.

5. Bottom line

1) Initial fluid resuscitation is still important, but once markers start to improve, back off.

2) Keep glucose < 200, but don't do tight control.

3) Give low-dose hydrocortisone to patients with refractory septic shock.

4) Norepinephrine is as good of a vasopressor as we have.

Authors: John Greenwood, Mike Winters, Haney Mallemat

危
重
病

67. 近5年内改变我们临床实践的危重病学文献

1. 成人呼吸窘迫综合征的液体治疗

1) 在第7天，接受保守（"干"）液体治疗的患者恢复得更好。

2) 虽然死亡率相同，但在下列几方面有差别：

(1) 氧浓度；

(2) 平台压；

(3) 机械通气时间；

(4) ICU住院时间。

3) 放置肺动脉导管还是中心静脉置管？

4) 在急诊科，仍要进行液体复苏，但一旦低血压和各脏器功能改善，就要减少液体摄入（目标是量出为入，维持 CVP=4）。

2. 血糖控制（允许轻度高血糖）

1) 与传统控制（低于 180 mg/dL）相比，严格控制（81 mg/dL～108 mg/dL）会使严重低血糖发生率增高并预后较差。

2) 血糖过高（超过 200 mg/dL）不好，但过低更坏。

3) 需要胰岛素时，要持续静脉滴注，不要静脉推注。

3. 感染性休克时的激素应用

1) 很明确的是，大剂量的激素使预后恶化。

2) 低剂量激素可缩短休克时间，但总的来说，并不改善28天死亡率，并可增加继发性感染的机会。

3) 不要对所有患者使用。

4) 建议应用于顽固性休克，对液体或升压药无反应者（50 mg 氢化可的松静脉注射，然后以 200 mg/24 h 持续滴注）。

5) 应该在1～2小时内见效。

4. 升压药在休克中的应用

1) 作为第二线升压药，应用垂体后叶素和去甲肾上腺素在死亡率方面无区别

2) 多巴胺作为第一线开压药与去甲肾上腺素比较。

3) 28天死亡率无差别。

4) 使用多巴胺的患者心律失常发生率较高。

5）对心源性休克患者，多巴胺可增加死亡率。

5. 要点

1）早期液体复苏是很重要的，但一旦指标好转，要减量。

2）维持血糖低于 200 mg/dL，但不要控制太严格。

3）小剂量的氢化可的松可用于顽固性感染性休克的患者。

4）升压可用去甲肾上腺素。

参考文献：

Diaz-Guzman E, Sanchez J, Arroliga AC. Updates in intensive care medicine：Studies that challenged our practice in the last 5 years. Cleveland Clini Med；2011，78(10)：665 – 674.

作者：John Greenwood，Mike Winters，Haney Mallemat

危
重
病

68. High-Yield Pearls for the ICU Patient in the ED

1. Increased mortality for ICU patients boarding in the Emergency Department; the increase is 1.5% per each hour of delayed transfer.

2. Intubated patients should receive analgesia BEFORE sedation; fentanyl is recommended because hemodynamically stable, but you can use anything. Good analgesia will also reduce total sedative dosing.

3. Use continuous capnography for the intubated patient; can detect equipment malfunction and allow titration of ventilation.

4. Keep an eye out for abdominal compartment syndrome. Physical exam is not always conclusive, should obtain bladder pressures.

5. Reduce the risk of ventilator-associated pneumonia by keeping endotracheal cuff pressures adequate and keeping the head of bed elevated 30 – 45 degrees.

Author: Haney Mallemat

美
国
急
诊
临
床
必
知
200
招

68. 急诊 ICU 患者处理的几个要点

1. 急诊科 ICU 患者每延迟 1 小时转到 ICU，其死亡率将增加 1.5%。

2. 气管插管的患者应该在用镇静药前镇痛，首选芬太尼，因为它对血流动力学影响小，当然也可以使用其他药物。良好的镇痛效果也将减少镇静药的总量。

3. 对气管插管的患者使用连续二氧化碳监测，可以发现设备故障，并调节呼吸机。

4. 要警惕腹腔筋膜室综合征。体检有时难以明确，应监测膀胱压力。

5. 为减少呼吸机相关性肺炎的风险，要保持充足的气管导管囊压力并保持床头抬高 30°~45°。

作者：Haney Mallemat

69. Critical Care Quickies?

1. High flow nasal cannula

Heated & humidified.

Can deliver almost 100% FiO_2.

20 – 50 L/min (some devices up to 60 L/min).

Enhances washout of nasopharyngeal "deadspace", reducing CO_2 re-breathing, improving oxygenation.

Provides ~3 – 6 cm/H_2O PEEP.

Increasing body of literature (observational) to support

2. Vascular access in crashing patient

1) Intraosseous access

(1) Very few contraindications (proximal fracture, hardware, vascular injury, o-verlying skin infection).

(2) Sites: Proximal tibia (>90% 1st attempt success rate); Humerus; Distal femur; Distal radius; and Medial malleolus.

(3) Can infuse any medication (except adenosine) or drip.

(4) Use 2% lidocaine w/o epi (1 – 2 mL followed by 10mL saline flush) to improve tolerance in a responsive patient.

2) Central line

(1) Ultrasound for subclavian.

(2) Higher success rate, fewer attempts, see http://ultrarounds.com/Ultra-rounds/Subclavian_Ultrasound.html.

(3) How bad is the femoral, really?

①Femoral vs. subclavian—no difference in infection rates.

②Femoral vs. IJ—lower rates for IJ.

③Externally rotating the leg increases diameter of femoral vein and brings it closer to the skin.

3. Bougie-aided cricothyrotomy

Vertical incision through skin, blunt dissection, horizontal incision through cricothyroid membrane.

Feed coude tip of bougie through cricothyroid membrane caudally.

Slide ET tube over bougie.

May take <1 minute!

4. Needle decompression for tension pneumothorax

1)2nd intercostal space, mid-clavicular line frequently fails!

2)5th intercostal space, anterior-axillary line being used more frequently

5. Ultrasound in cardiac arrest

Absence of cardiac motion on cardiac echo cannot be used as the sole determinant of when to stop resuscitation

Author: Mike Winters, MD

危
重
病

69. 危重病热题解答

1. 高流量鼻导管

加热和加湿；可提供几乎 100% 的氧浓度；20 ~ 50 L/min（某些设备可达 60 L/min）；增强鼻咽部"死腔"的排出，减少二氧化碳再吸入，改善氧合；提供 3 ~ 6 cm/H_2O PEEP；越来越多的文献（观察性）支持其使用。

2. 急救患者的血管通路

1）骨髓内针

（1）禁忌证很少（近端骨折、金属固定、血管损伤、局部皮肤感染）。

（2）穿刺部位：胫骨近端（第一次尝试的成功率 >90%）、肱骨、股骨远端、桡骨远端及内踝。

（3）可以注入或滴注所有药物（腺苷除外）。

（4）如患者神志清楚，可用 2% 不含肾上腺素的利多卡因（1 ~ 2 mL，然后用 10 mL 生理盐水冲洗），以改善患者的耐受性。

2）中心静脉置管

（1）超声直视下锁骨下静脉置管

成功率较高，减少穿刺次数，详见 http：//ultrarounds. com/Ultrarounds/Sub-clavian_Ultrasound. html。

（2）股静脉穿刺不好，真的吗？

①股静脉 vs. 锁骨下静脉——感染率无明显差别；

②股静脉 vs. 颈内静脉——颈内静脉感染率较低；

③将腿向外稍作旋转可增加股静脉直径并可使其更接近皮肤。

3. 探条辅助环甲膜切开

垂直切开皮肤，钝性分离，横向切开环甲膜；将探条尖尾端向脚方向通过环甲膜；将气管导管通过探条插入；可能在 1 分钟内可完成以上操作！

4. 张力性气胸的穿刺减压

1）第 2 肋间，锁骨中线穿刺经常失败！

2）第 5 肋间，腋前线被更频繁地使用。

5. 超声在心脏骤停时的应用

心脏超声显示没有心脏运动不能用来作为决定是否停止复苏的唯一指征。

参考文献:

1. Critical Care Medicine, 2011, 39(7)1607 – 1612.

2. Critical Care Medicine, 2012, 40(8): 2479 – 8524.

3. Emergency Medicine Australasia, 2012, 24(4): 408 – 413.

4. Air Medical Journal, 2009, 28(40): 191 – 194.

5. Academic Emergency Medicine, 2010, 17(6): 666 – 669.

6. Trauma-Injury Inf & Critical Care, 2011, 71(5): 1099 – 1103.

7. Archives of Surgery, 2012, 147(9): 813 – 881.

8. Trauma & Acute Care Surgery, 2012, 73(6): 1412 – 1417.

9. Academic Emergency Medicine, 2012, 19(10): 1119 – 1126.

作者: **Mike Winters, MD**

危
重
病

70. Hemodynamic Pearls from the 2013 Surviving Sepsis Guideline

1. The updated Surviving Sepsis Guidelines have been released and here are some recommendations as they pertain to hemodynamic management (grades of recommendations in parenthesis).

2. Fluid therapy

1) An initial fluid bolus of at least 30 mL/kg is recommended; crystalloids should be the initial fluids (1B).

2) Consider albumin when "substantial" amounts of crystalloid have been given (2C).

3) Use of hydroxyethyl starch is not recommended (1B).

3. Vasopressors (targeting MAP of at least 65 mmHg)

1) Norepinephrine (NE) is the vasopressor of choice (1B).

2) Epinephrine (EPI) if an additional agent is required; can be added to or substituted for NE (2B).

3) Vasopressin (0. 03 units/minute) can be added to NE; it should not be titrated or used as a single agent (ungraded).

4) In selected patients (e. g. , bradycardia or low-risk of tachyarrhythmia), dopamine may be considered (2C). Low-dose dopamine (for renal protection) should not be used (1A).

5) Phenylephrine (PE) is not recommended, except if (1C):

(1) Serious NE associated arrhythmias.

(2) Cardiac output can be measured and is increased with low MAP (PE can reduce cardiac output).

(3) Other therapies cannot achieve the target MAP.

4. Corticosteroids

1) Use if fluids and vasopressors cannot restore adequate perfusion.

2) Total daily dose of 200 mg (2C) administered by continuous infusion (2D).

3) ACTH stimulation test is not recommended (2B).

4) Tapering hydrocortisone when vasopressors have been discontinued (2D).

5. Inotropic therapy

Administer dobutamine if it is believed that cardiac filling pressures are elevated, cardiac output is low, or persistent signs of hypoperfusion despite other therapies (1C).

Author: Haney Mallemat

美国急诊临床必知200招

70. 2013年脓毒症急救指南的血液动力学要素

1. 新一版的脓毒症急救指南已出炉，这里是有关血液动力学方面的几个建议：

2. 液体治疗

1)建议最初的液体复苏的量为每公斤质量 30 mL，首选的液体应该是晶体液(1B)。

2)在输入相当量的晶体液后，要考虑给白蛋白(2C)。

3)不建议使用羟乙基淀粉液(1B)。

3. 应用升压药(目标 MAP 最低要达到 65 mmHg)

1)首选去甲肾上腺素(NE)(1B)。

2)如需要另外一种升压药，可加用肾上腺素(EPI)或取代 NE(2B)。

3)脑垂体后叶素(0.03 U/min)可与 NE 同用，但不要静脉滴注或单独使用。

4)在某些特定患者(如心动过缓或心动过速可能性不大)中，可考虑用多巴胺(2C)。不要用小剂量(肾保护剂量)的多巴胺(1A)。

5)不建议用去氧肾上腺素(新福林，PE)，除非以下情况(1C)：

(1)NE 导致严重心律失常。

(2)可监测心输出量，心输出量高但平均动脉压低(PE 可以降低心输出量)。

(3)其他方法无法维持理想的平均动脉压

4. 激素

1)如液体和升压药不能恢复正常循环时，可考虑使用。

2)总剂量为每天 200 mg(2C)，静脉持续滴注(2D)。

3)没有必要做 ACTH 刺激试验(2B)。

4)在停用升压药后，逐渐减少氢化可的松的用量(2D)。

5. 强心治疗

在如下的情况下可考虑使用多巴酚丁胺：心脏充盈压高，心输出量低，或其他治疗无效的持续性低灌注症状。

参考文献：

Surviving Sepsis Campaign: International Guidelines for Management of Severe Sepsis and Septic Shock. Crit Care Med, 2013, 41(2): 580 – 637.

作者：**Haney Mallemat**

危
重
病

71. Other Than Hemodynamic Pearls from the 2013 Surviving Sepsis Guideline

1. Antibiotics

Early and rapid resuscitation during the first 6 h (1C); blood cultures before antibiotic therapy (1C); broad-spectrum antimicrobials within 1 h of septic shock (1B) and severe sepsis without septic shock (1C) as the goal of therapy.

2. Hemoglobin

Hemoglobin target of $7-9$ g/dL in the absence of tissue hypoperfusion, ischemic coronary artery disease, or acute hemorrhage (1B).

3. Mechanical ventilation

Low tidal volume (1A) and inspiratory plateau pressure (1B) for acute respiratory distress syndrome (ARDS); application of at least a minimal amount of positive end-expiratory pressure (PEEP) in ARDS (1B); higher rather than lower level of PEEP for patients with sepsis-induced moderate or severe ARDS (2C); recruitment maneuvers in sepsis patients with severe refractory hypoxemia due to ARDS (2C); prone positioning in sepsis-induced ARDS patients with a PaO_2/FiO_2 ratio of $\leqslant 100$ mm Hg (2C); head-of-bed elevation in mechanically ventilated patients unless contraindicated (1B).

4. Fluid resuscitation

A conservative fluid strategy for patients with established ARDS who do not have evidence of tissue hypoperfusion (1C).

5. IV sedation

Protocols for weaning and sedation (1A); minimizing use of either intermittent bolus sedation or continuous infusion sedation targeting specific titration endpoints (1B).

6. Neuromuscular blockers

Avoidance of neuromuscular blockers if possible in the septic patient without ARDS (1C); a short course of neuromuscular blocker (no longer than 48 h) for patients with early ARDS and a $PaO_2/FiO_2 < 150$ mm Hg (2C).

7. Insulin

Starting insulin when two consecutive blood glucose levels are > 180 mg/dL, targeting an upper blood glucose $\leqslant 180$ mg/dL (1A).

Author: Feng Xiao

71. 2013 年国际脓毒症急救指南 除血液动力学以外的要素

1. 抗生素

第一个 6 h 内的早期和快速的复苏(1C);给抗生素前要做血培养(1C);治疗的目标是在脓毒性休克(1B)或严重脓毒症没有休克(1C)1 h 内给广谱抗生素。

2. 血红蛋白

在没有组织低灌注、缺血性冠状动脉疾病或急性出血的情况下,保持血红蛋白在 7 ~ 9 g/dL(1B)。

3. 呼吸机

对急性呼吸窘迫综合征(ARDS)患者要用低潮气量(1A),低吸气平台压(1B),和最小的 PEEP(1B);对脓毒症导致的中重度 ARDS 患者要用稍高的 PEEP(2C);对由 ARDS 造成顽固性低氧的脓毒症患者可采用肺复张手法(2C);如脓毒症 ARDS 患者 $PaCO_2/FiO_2 < 100$ mmHg,可将患者置俯卧位(2C);如没有禁忌证,可将机械通气患者的床头抬高(1B)。

4. 液体复苏

对没有组织低灌注迹象的 ARDS 患者,液体复苏趋于保守(IC)。

5. 静脉镇静药

要建立停止呼吸机和镇静的方案(1A);设定具体的指标来限制间歇性静脉注射或持续静脉滴注镇静药的使用(1B)。

6. 神经肌肉阻滞药

对没有 ARDS 的脓毒症患者,尽量不要用神经肌肉阻滞药(1C);如患者出现早期 ARDS 并 $PaO_2/FiO_2 < 150$ mmHg,可考虑短期应用(不超过48 h)神经肌肉阻滞药(2C)。

7. 胰岛素

如连续两次测量血糖水平超过 180 mg/dL,要开始使用胰岛素,保持最高血糖≤180 mg/dL(1A)。

参考文献:

Surviving Sepsis Campaign: International Guidelines for Management of Severe Sepsis and Septic Shock. Crit Care Med, 2013, 41(2): 580 – 637.

作者: Feng Xiao

危重病

72. Blood pressure and organ perfusion

Which patient has a better blood pressure, the patient with a blood pressure of 110/40 mmHg or the patient with a blood pressure of 90/60 mmHg?

1. Mean arterial pressure (MAP) is generally considered to be the organ perfusion pressure in an individual. Because MAP requires an inconvenient calculation, we've all been taught... misled perhaps... into focusing on systolic blood pressure (SBP) as a marker of how well-perfused a patient is, and we tend to ignore the diastolic blood pressure (DBP).

2. It's important to remember, however, that we spend most of our lives in diastole, not systole. As a result, our organs spend more time being perfused during diastole than systole. The MAP takes this into account: MAP = (SBP + DBP + DBP)/3. DBP is more important than SBP!

3. So which patient is perfusing his vital organs better, the one with a BP of 110/40 or the one with a BP of 90/60 mmHg? Do the MAP calculation... 90/60 mmHg is better than 110/40 mmHg!

4. Pay more attention to those diastolic BPs!

Author: Amal Mattu

72. 血压和器官灌注

血压 110/40 mmHg 或血压 90/60 mmHg,哪种情况要好些呢?

1. 对个体而言,平均动脉压(MAP)一般被认为是器官灌注压。MAP 需要计算得出,由于我们在过去所学到的(也可能是被误导),收缩压(SBP)是评定一个患者灌注好坏的指标,以至我们经常忽视了舒张压(DBP)。

2. 但是,一定要记住,在我们一生中,是舒张期而不是收缩期所占用的时间更多。也就是说,我们各个脏器在舒张期得到灌注的时间要比收缩期多得多。在 MAP 的计算中对这个问题也有所考虑:MAP =(SBP + DBP + DBP)/3。DBP 要比 SBP 重要!

3. 这样,哪一种状态对患者脏器灌注更有效,是血压为 110/40 mmHg,还是血压为 90/60 mmHg? 算一下 MAP……90/60 mmHg 要好于 110/40 mmHg!

4. 要多留意舒张压!

作者:Amal Mattu

73. Can your breath predict fluid responsiveness?

1. Fluid boluses are often administered to patients in shock as a first-line intervention to increase cardiac output. Previous literature states, however, that only 50% of patients in shock will respond to a fluid bolus.

2. Several validated techniques exist to distinguish which patients will respond to a fluid bolus and which will not; one method is the passive leg raise (PLR) maneuver. A drawback to PLR is that it requires direct measurement of cardiac output, either by invasive hemodynamic monitoring or using advanced bedside ultrasound techniques.

3. Another technique to quantify changes in cardiac output is through measurement of end-tidal CO_2 ($ETCO_2$). The benefits of measuring $ETCO_2$ is that it can be continuously measured and can be performed non-invasively on mechanically ventilated patients.

4. A 5% or greater increase in $ETCO_2$ following a PLR maneuver has been found to be a good predictor of fluid responsiveness with reliability similar to invasive measures.

Author: Haney Mallemat

73. 你的呼吸能够预测对液体复苏的反应吗？

1. 作为第一线的增加心输出量治疗措施，休克患者经常接受快速静脉输液。然而，过去的文献显示，只有50%的休克患者会对快速液体输注有反应

2. 有几个已被证实的方法能够区分哪些患者会对快速液体输注有反应，哪些患者不会有反应。其中的一个办法是被动抬腿试验（PLR）。PLR试验的一个缺点是，它需要通过侵入性血流动力学监测或使用高级的床旁超声技术直接测量心输出量。

3. 另一种可以反应心输出量改变的指标是测量潮气末二氧化碳（$ETCO_2$）。测量 $ETCO_2$ 的好处是，它可以连续地监测，并可以非侵入性地在机械通气患者中使用。

4. 在 PLR 后超过5%的 $ETCO_2$ 增加已被证实是一个与侵入性措施同样可靠的预测对液体复苏反应程度的指标。

参考文献：

Monnet, X. et al. End-tidal carbon dioxide is better than arterial pressure for predicting volume responsiveness by the passive leg raising test. Intensive Care Med, 2013, 39(1): 93 - 100.

作者：**Haney Mallemat**

危重病

74. The effects of HES

1. A study by Perner, et al recently published in NEJM observed that using hydroxyethyl starch (HES) as a resuscitation fluid increased mortality and renal replacement therapy at 90 days as compared to lactated acetate.

2. Another recent trial, called the "Crystalloid versus Hydroxyethyl Starch Trial" (CHEST) was a prospective randomized control trial from Australia comparing the use of 6% HES and 0.9% sodium chloride as a resuscitation fluid in the critically ill.

3. With 7,000 patients enrolled (3,500 in each group), the CHEST trial is the largest single-trial of HES to date; the primary outcome was 90 – day mortality and secondary outcomes were acute kidney injury (AKI) and renal-replacement therapy.

4. The study concluded that there were no significant risks in morality or renal failure between groups, but significantly more patients in the HES group required renal replacement therapy.

5. Bottom line: There is still no convincing data that patients receiving HES as part of their resuscitation have better outcomes compared to crystalloid (normal saline or lactated ringers) and there is increased harm with their use. Furthermore, the increased cost of HES does not appear to justify their routine use.

Author: Haney Mallemat

美
国
急
诊
临
床
必
知
200
招

74. 羟乙基淀粉液(HES)的作用

1. Perner 等最近在《新英格兰医学杂志》(NEJM)上发表了一篇有关羟乙基淀粉液(HES)在液体复苏中的应用的论文。该研究发现：与乳酸乙酯液相比，HES增加了患者 90 天内的死亡率和需行肾脏替代治疗的患者人数。

2. 另外，最近一项被称为"晶体和羟乙基淀粉液试验(CHEST)"的来自澳大利亚的前瞻性随机对照临床试验，对 6% HES 与 0.9% 氯化钠在危重患者液体复苏中的应用进行了比较。

3. CHEST 研究包括了 7,000 位患者(每组有 3,500 人)，是目前有关 HES 临床应用的最大项目。主要的预后标准是 90 天死亡率，另一个标准是急性肾损伤和需行肾替代治疗。

4. 此研究结果显示两者在死亡率和肾衰竭方面没有差别，但在 HES 组需肾替代治疗的患者有明显增加。

5. 要点

还没有有利数据支持在液体复苏时使用 HES 比晶体液(生理盐水或乳酸林格氏液)预后更好。另外，HES 的昂贵价格也限制了它在临床上的常规应用。

参考文献：

Perner A., et al. Hydroxyethyl Starch 130/0.4 versus Ringer's Acetate in Severe Sepsis, N Engl J Med, 2012, 27.

MyBurgh J. Hydroxyethyl Starch or Saline for Fluid Resuscitation in Intensive Care. N Engl J Med, 2012, 17.

作者：**Haney Mallemat**

75. More Bad News for HES

1. Hydroxyethyl starch (HES) is a colloid used for volume resuscitation in critically-ill patients.

2. Previous studies have compared crystalloids to HES during fluid resuscitation and have demonstrated that HES has an increased cost with more adverse effects. Adverse effects may include:

1) Coagulopathy.

2) Acute kidney injury.

3) Increased mortality.

3. In the United States, the Federal Drug Administration published a warning on June 24th 2013 with respect to the use of HES in critically ill adult patients. Specifically, it warned about the use of HES in patients.

1) with sepsis.

2) with pre-existing kidney injury.

3) admitted to the ICU.

4) undergoing heart surgery with cardiopulmonary bypass.

4. If a decision to use HES is made, the FDA warning advises to:

1) discontinue use of HES at the first sign of renal injury or coagulopathy.

2) continue to monitor renal function for at least 90 days (all patients).

5. Bottom line: With an increased cost and evidence of harm compared to crystalloids, it appears the indications for use of HES are rapidly declining.

Author: Haney Mallemat

75. 更多的有关 HES 的坏消息

1. 羟乙基淀粉(HES)是用于病危患者容量复苏的一种胶体。

2. 以往的研究对晶体液和 HES 在液体复苏中的应用进行了比较,发现 HES 不但成本高而且不良反应多。其不良反应包括:

1) 凝血功能障碍;

2) 急性肾损伤;

3) 死亡率增加。

3. 在美国,联邦药物管理局(FDA)在 2013 年 6 月 24 日发表了一份有关危重成人患者使用 HES 的警告。这个警告明确警示在下列患者中要小心应用 HES:

1) 脓毒症;

2) 已有肾损伤;

3) ICU 病房患者;

4) 体外循环心脏手术。

4. 如果决定使用 HES,FDA 的警告建议:

1) 如果出现肾损伤或凝血功能障碍的迹象要停止使用 HES;

2) 至少要继续监测肾功能 90 d(所有患者)。

5. 要点

与晶体液相比,HES 成本高并有更多的有害证据,它的使用适应证正在迅速减少。

参考文献:

Perner A, et al. Hydroxyethyl Starch 130/0. 4 versus Ringer's Acetate in Severe Sepsis. N Engl J Med, 2012 Jun 27.

MyBurgh, J. Hydroxyethyl Starch or Saline for Fluid Resuscitation in Intensive Care, N Engl J Med, 2012, 17.

作者: Haney Mallemat

危重病

76. Too much salt may NOT be sweet

1. Previous pearls have described the increasing evidence against colloid (e. g. , hydroxyethyl starch) use during resuscitation. Now it appears that the crystalloid 0.9% normal saline (NS) may be under fire.

2. The use of large volumes of NS has been associated with hyperchloremic metabolic acidosis and harm in animal studies. The risk of harm in humans, however, has been less clear.

3. Bellomo et al. conducted a prospective observational study in which patients being resuscitated in the control group received NS at the clinicians' discretion; i. e. , chloride-liberal strategy. The use of NS was restricted in the intervention group, where other less chloride containing fluids were used for resuscitation (e. g. , Ringer's Lactate); i. e. , a chloride-restrictive strategy.

4. The authors found that when compared to patients in the chloride-liberal group, the chloride-restrictive group had significantly less rise in baseline creatinine, less overall AKI, and a reduced need for renal replacement therapy.

5. Bottom line: Although this was only an observational study, the liberal use of normal saline during resuscitation may increase the risk of AKI and renal replacement therapy.

Author: **Haney Mallemat**

76. 生理盐水在复苏中的作用

1. 在前面的必知里介绍了没有证据支持胶体液(羟乙基淀粉液, HES)在液体复苏中的作用。现在看来, 晶体液(0.9%生理盐水, NS)的应用也有下降趋势。

2. 动物实验显示：大量生理盐水的使用与高氯性代谢性酸中毒有关, 并造成危害。但是, 它对人体的损害还不清楚。

3. Bellomo 等进行了一项前瞻性观察研究, 对照组的患者根据病情的需要接受生理盐水(氯随意方案)；治疗组的患者接受含氯浓度低的复苏液(乳酸林格氏液, 氯限制方案)。

4. 作者发现：与氯随意方案组患者比, 氯限制组患者的基础肌酐水平增加明显减低, 急性肾损伤发生率和对肾替代治疗的需要也有所减低。

5. 要点

虽然这只是一个观察性报告, 但它提示在液体复苏时生理盐水的大量应用, 会增加急性肾损伤和肾替代治疗的风险。

参考文献：

Bellomo, R. et al. Association between a chloride-liberal vs. chloride-restrictive intravenous fluid administration strategy and kidney injury in critically ill adults. JAMA, 2012, 308(15)：1566 – 1572. doi：10. 1001/jama. 2012. 13356.

作者：Haney Mallemat

危
重
病

77. Delirium in the Critically Ⅲ?

1. Delirium has been shown to be an independent predictor of mortality and can occur in up to 75% of critically ill patients.

2. Whether preventing or treating delirium in the critically ill patient, consider the
following:

1) Minimize the use of anticholinergic medications (i. e. diphenhydramine, chlor-
promazine).

2) Ensure pain is adequately controlled (avoid meperidine and tramadol).

3) Be careful with sedative medications; consider bolus dosing and daily interruption of continuous infusions.

4) Additional measures to treat delirious patients include reducing sensory depriva-
tion, promoting normal sleep-wake cycles, early physical rehabilitation, and treating
psychosis.

Author: Michael Winters

77. 危重患者的谵妄表现

1. 已有证据证实：谵妄是一个预测死亡率增加的独立危险因素，可出现在 75% 的危重患者身上。

2. 预防或治疗谵妄的危重患者时，要考虑如下情况：

1）限制抗胆碱能药物的使用（如苯海拉明、氯丙嗪）；

2）有效控制疼痛（避免杜冷丁、曲马多）；

3）小心使用镇静剂，可用静脉推注，对持续注射的药物每天要有间隔时间；

4）治疗谵妄患者的其他办法包括：减少感官剥夺，建立正常的睡眠规律，早期物理康复和治疗精神紊乱。

参考文献：

Bienvenu OJ, Neufeld KJ, Needham DM. Treatment of four psychiatric emergencies in the intensive care unit. Crit Care Med, 2012, 40: 2662 – 2670.

作者：**Michael Winters**

危
重
病

78. Pediatric Pearls from the 2013 Surviving Sepsis Guideline

1. Oxygenation and ventilation

Therapy with face mask oxygen, high flow nasal cannula oxygen, or nasopharyngeal continuous PEEP in the presence of respiratory distress and hypoxemia (2C), use of physical examination therapeutic endpoints such as capillary refill (2C).

2. Fluid therapy

For septic shock associated with hypovolemia, the use of crystalloids or albumin to deliver a bolus of 20 mL/kg of crystalloids (or albumin equivalent) over 5 to 10 mins (2C).

3. Inotropes and vasodilators

More common use of inotropes and vasodilators for low cardiac output septic shock associated with elevated systemic vascular resistance (2C).

4. Corticosteroids

Use of hydrocortisone only in children with suspected or proven "absolute"' adrenal insufficiency (2C).

Author: Feng Xiao

78. 2013 年国际脓毒症急救指南中有关儿科患者的要点

1. 供氧和通气

在呼吸困难和低氧血症发生的情况下，可用面罩给氧、高流量鼻导管给氧或鼻咽部持续 PEEP 给氧(2C)。使用体征如毛细血管再充盈时间(2C)作为观察效果的指标。

2. 液体治疗

感染性休克的低血容量，可在 5～10 min 内给晶体(20 mL/kg)或等量的白蛋白(2C)。

3. 强心药和血管舒张药

对伴有周围血管阻力增加和低心输出量的感染性休克患者常用强心药和血管舒张药(2C)。

4. 激素

对于儿童，只有在怀疑或确定有"绝对"肾上腺皮质功能不全时，才考虑使用氢化可的松(2C)。

参考文献：

Surviving Sepsis Campaign: International Guidelines for Management of Severe Sepsis and Septic Shock. Crit Care Med, 2013, 41(2): 580 – 637.

作者：Feng Xiao

危
重
病

79. Jennifer Guyther

1. Passive leg raise (PLR) has been studied in adults as a bedside tool to predict volume responsiveness. Can this be applied to children?

2. A single center prospective study looked at 40 intensive care patients ranging in age from 1 month to 12.5 years. They used a noninvasive monitoring system that could measure heart rate, stroke volume and cardiac output

3. These parameters were measured at a baseline, after PLR, after another baseline and after a 10 mL/kg bolus.

4. Overall, changes in the cardiac index varied with PLR. However, there was a statistically significant correlation in children over 5 years showing an increase in cardiac index with PLR and with a fluid bolus.

5. Bottom line: In children older than 5 years, PLR can be a quick bedside tool to assess for fluid responsiveness, especially if worried about fluid overload and in an under served area.

Author: Jennifer Guyther

79. 儿童被动抬腿试验

1. 被动抬腿(PLR)试验已经在成人中被用作床旁预测容量反应的方法。但这种试验方法适用于儿童吗?

2. 一个单中心、前瞻性研究观察了 40 位年龄 1 个月至 12.5 岁的重症监护患者。他们使用了一种非侵入性的监测系统,可以测量心率、每搏输出量和心输出量。

3. 这些参数的测量点为:基点、PLR 后、回到基线和 10 mL/kg 静脉注射(生理盐水)后。

4. 总体而言,心脏指数随 PLR 结果改变而变化。然而,5 岁以上儿童心脏指数因 PLR 结果和扩容的变化有统计学意义。

5. 要点

对 5 岁以上的儿童,PLR 可以作为快速评估输液反应的床旁手段,尤其是在担心液体超负荷时或在医疗条件差的地区。

参考文献:

Lu et al. The Passive Leg Raise Test to Predict Fluid Responsiveness in Children-Preliminary Observations. Indian J Pediatr, 2013, (epub ahead of print).

作者: Jennifer Guyther

危
重
病

80. Lactate use in the pediatric emergency department

1. Lactate is commonly used in the adult ED when evaluating septic patients, but there is a lack of literature validating its use in the pediatric ED. Pediatric studies have suggested that in the ICU population, elevated lactate is a predictor of mortality and may be the earliest marker of death.

2. A retrospective chart review over a 1 year period showed that one elevated serum lactate correlated with increased pulse, respiratory rate, white blood cell count and platelets. Serum lactate had a negative correlation with BUN, serum bicarbonate and age.

3. Elevated lactate levels were higher for admitted patients. However, the mean serum lactate level was not statistically different between those diagnosed with sepsis and those that were not. The study included 289 patients less then 18 years who had both blood cultures and lactate drawn.

4. This community hospital had a sepsis protocol in place that automatically ordered a lactate with blood cultures. Only previously healthy children were included. The study is limited by its small sample size and overall low lactate levels.

5. Despite having a protocol in place, only 39% of patients who had blood cultures drawn and had lactate levels available for analysis. The mean serum lactate in this study was 2.04 mM indicating that the study population may not have been sick enough to determine mortality implications. There were no serial measurements.

6. Bottom line: Consider measuring serum lactate in your pediatric patient with suspected sepsis. Pediatric ICU literature does suggest that a serum lactate as low as 3 mM is associated with an increased mortality in the ICU.

Author: Jennifer Guyther

美国急诊临床必知200招

80. 乳酸水平在儿科急诊中的应用

1. 在急诊科乳酸通常用于成人脓毒症患者的评估，但其在儿科急诊中的应用却缺乏文献资料。儿科的研究表明，在 ICU 患者中，乳酸升高是预测死亡的一个指标，可能是一个最早的预测死亡的标志。

2. 一项超过 1 年的回顾性研究显示：高血清乳酸与增加的脉搏、呼吸频率、白细胞计数和血小板有关。但血清乳酸与 BUN、血清碳酸氢钠和年龄呈负相关。

3. 住院患者的乳酸水平较高。然而，确诊为脓毒症患者的平均血清乳酸水平与非脓毒症患者之间的差异无统计学意义。该研究纳入了 289 例 18 岁以下并做了血培养和乳酸测定的患者。

4. 这个私立医院有一个常规的脓毒症治疗方案，会自动检测乳酸和血培养。研究只纳入了既往健康的儿童。这项研究的缺陷为小样本和乳酸水平低。

5. 尽管有常规治疗方案，仍只有 39% 的患者有血培养和乳酸水平的结果可用于分析。这项研究的平均血清乳酸为 2.04 mmol/L，表明这些患者的病情并没有严重到需要判断死亡率。同时，该研究没有对乳酸进行连续测量。

6. 要点

对疑似脓毒症儿科的患者，要考虑检测血清乳酸水平。文献表明：在儿科 ICU，即使 3 mmol/L 的血清乳酸也与 ICU 死亡率增加有关。

参考文献：

Reed et al. Serum Lactate as a Screening Tool and Predictor of Outcome in Pediatric Patients Presenting to the Emergency Department With Suspected Infection. Pediatric Emergency Care, 2013, 29: 787－791.

作者：Jennifer Guyther

危重病

81. Pediatric HHS: Becoming More Frequent

1. Emergency Physicians should be aware that hyperglycemic hyperosmolar state (HHS) occurs in children and that HHS is likely to become more common given the increasing incidence of childhood obesity and type 2 DM. Furthermore, HHS, although classically associated with type 2 DM, has also been reported increasingly with type 1 DM.

2. Correctly differentiating HHS vs. DKA is crucial as treatment principles are different.

Clinically, HHS and DKA differ by the severity of dehydration and whether or not ketosis and metabolic acidosis are present.

3. HHS is characterized by the triad of hyperglycemia (typically > 600 mg/dL), hyperosmolality (serum osmolality > 320 mOsm/L), and absence of significant acidosis or ketosis.

4. Fluid therapy is the cornerstone of management of pediatric HHS. Initial bolus of NaCl 20 mL/kg should be given and can be repeated until peripheral circulation/perfusion is established. Fluid deficits should then be gradually corrected over 48 h. Fluid administration alone results in a substantial decline in serum glucose.

5. Severe dehydration, electrolyte disturbance, and hypertonicity are far more frequent causes of death in HHS than is cerebral edema; therefore, concerns about cerebral edema should not deter the clinician from administering the necessary amount of fluid to restore adequate hydration and perfusion.

6. In general, insulin administration should be considered only when serum glucose concentrations are no longer declining adequately (< 50 mg/dL · h) with fluid administration alone or in children with significant ketosis and acidosis.

7. Unlike DKA, insulin therapy is usually not necessary for resolution of ketosis in HHS. Of note, some children with type 1 DM may have features of HHS (i. e. severe hyperglycemia), if high-carbohydrate-containing beverages have been used to quench thirst before presentation.

Author: Mimi Lu

81. 儿童高血糖高渗状态(HHS)会越来越常见

1. 急诊医师应该知道，高血糖高渗状态(HHS)可以发生在儿童，并且因为儿童肥胖和2型糖尿病发病率越来越高 HHS 可能更常见。此外，虽然一般认为 HHS 与2型糖尿病相关，但也有越来越多的报道认为 HSS 与1型糖尿病相关。

2. 正确区分 HHS 与糖尿病酮症酸中毒(DKA)至关重要，因为它们的治疗原则不同。临床上，HHS 和 DKA 的差别在于脱水的程度不同和是否存在酮症及代谢性酸中毒。

3. HHS 的特点是三联征：高血糖(通常 >600 mg/dL)、高渗(血浆渗透压 > 320 mOsm/L)和无明显的酸中毒或酮症。

4. 液体疗法是治疗小儿 HHS 的主要措施。最初要快速静脉注射 20 mL/kg 的生理盐水并可以反复进行，直至末梢循环/灌注重新建立。然后将全部所需液体在 48 h 内逐步输入。单靠输液就可使血糖大幅下降。

5. HHS 的严重脱水，电解质紊乱，高渗要比脑水肿造成更多的死亡。因此，不能因为担心发生脑水肿就不敢给患者补充恢复充足的水分和灌注的必要的液体量。

6. 在一般情况下，只有在充分补液后血糖浓度不再明显下降[<50 mg/(dL·h)]或儿童有明显酮症或酸中毒时才应考虑给胰岛素。

7. 与 DKA 不同的是，HHS 酮症的改善通常不需要胰岛素。值得注意的是，如果1型糖尿病儿童在就诊前喝了大量高碳水化合物饮料可以出现 HHS 的特征(如严重的高血糖)。

参考文献：

Arora R, Chiwane S, Hartwig E, et al. A Child with Altered Sensorium, Hyperglycemia, and Elevated Troponins. J Emerg Med, Epub July, 2013.

McDonnell CM, Pedreira CC, Vadamalayan B, et al. Diabetic ketoacidosis, hyperosmolarity and hypernatremia: are high-carbohydrate drinks worsening initial presentation?. Pediatr Diabetes, 2005, 6: 90 – 94.

Zeitler P, Haqq A, Rosenbloom A, et al. Hyperglycemic hyperosmolar syndrome in children: pathophysiological considerations and suggested guidelines for treatment. J Pediatr, 2011, 158: 9 – 14.

作者：**Mimi Lu**

危
重
病

82. Hypertonic saline-safe for transport?

1. Management of the patient with intracranial hypertension represents one of the most challenging situations the emergency physician faces. Doing so in a community setting when the patient is a child is even more daunting. But devising therapies that can safely be given while the patient is being transferred to a tertiary center for definitive therapy is truly critical.

2. Fortunately, a recent study suggests that 3% saline fits this bill nicely. Given the risk of vasconstriction with hyperventilation and the risk of hypovolemia with mannitol, hypertonic saline has emerged as beneficial therapy when trying to decrease intracranial pressure (ICP) in both children and adults.

3. In late 2011, the Loma Linda University Medical Center published a retrospective analysis of their experience using 3% saline during transport of children at risk of elevated ICPs. While they found the expected rise in electrolytes such as sodium, chloride and bicarbonate, importantly they found no adverse effects (such as "local effects, renal abnormalities or central pontine myelinolysis") related to the administration of hypertonic saline, even though 96% of patients received the infusion through a peripheral line.

4. Bottom line: Hypertonic saline appears to be a viable and safe option for use as therapy to decrease ICH during transport of children at risk for intracranial hypertension.

Author: Mimi Lu

82. 高张盐水——转运患儿时使用安全吗？

1. 处理颅内压增高是急诊医生面临的严峻挑战之一，在社区医院处理儿科患者时会更具危险性。因此制定一个能在将患者转移到上级医院途中安全使用的明确治疗方案尤为关键。

2. 幸运的是，一项新的临床研究提示 3% 的盐水可以满足这一要求。由于过度通气可能造成血管收缩而甘露醇可能造成低容量，高张盐水已成为降低儿童和成人颅内压的有效方法。

3. 2011 年末，罗马林达大学医学中心发表了一篇有关转运有颅高压危险儿童使用 3% 盐水的回顾性研究论文。虽然他们在电解质检测中发现了预料中的 Na^+、K^+、$NaHCO_3$ 增高，但没有发现与注射高张盐水有关的不良反应（如局部反应，肾功异常或脑桥中部髓鞘溶解），即使 96% 的患者是通过末梢血管接受注射的。

4. 要点

在转运有颅高压危险的儿童时，高张盐水是有效安全的降低颅内压的方法。

参考文献：

Luu JL, Wendtland CL, Gross MF, et al. Three percent saline administration during pediatric critical care transport. Ped Emerg Care, 2011, 27(12): 1113 – 1117.

作者: **Mimi Lu**

危
重
病

83. Propofol Infusion Syndrome (PRIS)

1. Propofol is generally a well-tolerated sedative/amnestic but occasionally it can lead to the propofol infusion syndrome (PRIS); a metabolic disorder causing end-organ dysfunction

2. Suspect PRIS in patients with increasing lactate levels, worsening metabolic acidosis, worsening renal function, increased triglyceride levels, or creatinine kinase levels. End-organ effects include:

1) Myocardial dysfunction/Arrhythmias.

2) Rhabdomyolysis.

3) Acute renal failure.

3. The true incidence of PRIS is unknown, however, certain risk factors have been identified:

1) Doses >4 – 5 mg/kg/hour.

2) <18 years of age.

3) Critically-ill patients; especially receiving vasopressors or steroids.

4) History of mitochondrial disorders.

5) Infusions >48 hours.

4. Prevent PRIS by using adequate analgesia (with morphine or fentanyl) post-intubation, which may reduce the overall dosage of propofol ultimately reducing the risk.

5. If PRIS develops, stop propofol and provide supportive care; IV fluids, ensuring good urine output, adequate oxygenation, dialysis (if indicated), vasopressor and inotropic support.

Author: Haney Mallemat

83.丙泊酚注射综合征

1.通常情况下，丙泊酚通常是一种耐受良好的镇静及帮助遗忘药物，但偶尔会造成所谓的丙泊酚注射综合征(PRIS)，即可导致器官功能衰竭的代谢紊乱。

2.如患者出现乳酸血症、代谢性酸中毒、肾功能恶化、甘油三酯水平增高，或肌酸激酶水平增高时，要怀疑PRIS。器官损伤包括：

1)心脏功能障碍/心律失常；

2)横纹肌溶解症；

3)急性肾功能衰竭。

3.虽然PRIS的确切发生率还不清楚，但其危险因素有：

1)使用剂量超过 4~5 mg/(kg·h)；

2)年龄在 18 岁以下；

3)危重患者(尤其是需要升压药或激素的患者)；

4)线粒体功能紊乱病史；

5)注射时间超过 48 h。

4.气管插管后用足量的止痛药(如吗啡或芬太尼)有助于减少丙泊酚的用量，进而降低发生 PRIS 的风险。

5.一旦发生 PRIS，就应该停止用丙泊酚并加强支持疗法，包括静脉输液，保证足够的尿量，吸氧，透析(如需要)，给予升压药和强心药。

作者：**Haney Mallemat**

84. VV-ECMO for Refractory Hypoxemia

1. In the absence of significant cardiac disease, patients with refractory hypoxic respiratory failure should be considered for venovenous extracorporeal membrane oxygenation (VV-ECMO).

2. Though indications vary slightly among organizations, the Extracorporeal Life Support Organization states that ECMO is indicated when the PaO_2/FiO_2 is < 80 mmHg on FiO_2 > 90% or safe plateau pressures (< 30 cmH_2O) cannot be maintained.

3. A few pearls when initiating VV-ECMO:

1) Fluids are often needed in the first few hours after initiation of ECMO.

2) Reduce tidal volumes to maintain plateau pressures < 25 cmH_2O.

3) Decrease FiO_2 to maintain oxygen saturations > 88%.

4) Use a hemoglobin threshold of 7 – 8 g/dL for blood transfusion.

Author: Michael Winters

84. 静脉静脉－体外膜肺氧合治疗顽固性缺氧

1. 在没有明显心脏疾病情况下，对顽固性缺氧性呼吸衰竭的患者，可考虑使用静脉静脉－体外膜肺氧合（VV-ECMO）

2. 虽然每个医疗机构的应用指征有所差异，但体外生命支持协会明确指出应用 ECMO 的指征包括吸入氧浓度（FiO_2）>90% 时，PaO_2/FiO_2 <80 mmHg；或不能够维持安全的平台压（低于 30 cmH_2O）。

3. 在开始使用 VV-ECMO 时一定要注意：

1）在前几个小时内，通常需要补充液体；

2）减低潮气量，维持平台压低于 25 cmH_2O；

3）降低 FiO_2，维持氧饱和度 >88% 即可；

4）血红蛋白低于 7 ~ 8 g/dL 时才考虑输血。

参考文献：

Combes A, et al. What is the niche for extracorporeal membrane oxygenation in severe acute respiratory distress syndrome? Curr Opin Crit Care, 2012, 18: 527 – 532.

作者：**Michael Winters**

危
重
病

85. Extracorporeal Membrane Oxygenation (ECMO) in 2012?

1. Venovenous ECMO (VV ECMO)

1) Started off being used in pediatric patients in the 1970's.

2) Now being used more for adults with reversible lung processes or as a bridge to lung transplant.

3) Only used as an oxygenator to give the lungs a break while it heals from its reversible process or while awaiting lung transplant.

4) A criteria for its use is that the patient must have a good intrinsic mechanical pump or heart.

2. Venoarterial ECMO (VA-ECMO)

1) Recently been used a lot more frequently and now something that is available for ED physicians.

2) Works similarly to VV-ECMO except that it also provides circulatory support.

3) Should be thought of as a way to give the heart and lungs a break from this reversible disease process.

4) Primary use is in refractory cardiogenic shock and should be considered early to get the most benefit.

5) Complications

(1) Limb ischemia.

(2) Artery laceration.

(3) Patients need to be anticoagulated.

3. End goal is to buy more time to PCI, CABG, or heart transplant.

4. Patients usually are on vasopressors but will not need them once on ECMO.

5. Could possibly be used in the community setting as a bridge to transport.

6. Use in cardiac arrest

1) A few small case studies show it is associated with good outcomes.

2) A very select population to consider its use.

(1) Relatively healthy.

(2) Short down times (<10 minutes).

(3) Should have a reversible cause to their cardiac arrest.

7. No risks for adverse outcomes from ECMO use.

Authors: Haney Mallemat, John Greenwood

85. 2012 年的体外膜肺氧合（ECMO）

1. 静脉静脉 - 体外膜肺氧合（VV-ECMO）

1）最初在 20 世纪 70 年代用于儿科患者；

2）现在多用于患有可逆性肺疾病或需要肺移植的成年患者；

3）只是作为人工肺给有可逆性病变的肺一段恢复的时间，或是用于等待肺移植的情况；

4）应用它的前提是患者一定要有一个好的内在机械泵（心脏）。

2. 静脉动脉 - 体外膜肺氧合（VA-ECMO）

1）近期应用相当多，也是现在急诊医生可以使用的治疗手段；

2）VA-ECMO 除了同时支持循环系统以外，其他与 VV-ECMO 相似；

3）作为给心和肺争取从可逆性病变恢复时间的一个方式；

4）主要用于顽固性心源性休克，为得到最好的效果，要尽早用。

5）合并症

（1）肢体缺血；

（2）动脉撕裂；

（3）患者需要抗凝。

3. 最终的目的是为经皮冠状动脉介入、冠状动脉搭桥或心脏移植争取时间。

4. 一旦用上 ECMO，患者就不再需要使用升压药。

5. 也可以在从社区医院向上级医院转运的患者中应用。

6. 在心脏骤停患者中的应用

1）只有几个小样本的研究结果表明，它的使用与良性预后有关；

2）仅在极少数人群适用；

（1）相对健康

（2）骤停时间短（少于 10 min）

（3）造成心脏骤停的原因是可逆的

7. ECMO 的使用不会造成恶性后果。

参考文献：

Peura JL, Colvin-Adams M, et al. Recommendations for the use of mechanical circulatory support: device strategies and patient selection. Circulation. 2012; 126: 2648 – 2667.

Sayer GT, Baker JN, Parks KA. Heart rescue: the role of mechanical circulatory support in the management of severe refractory cardiogenic shock. Curr Opin Crit Care, 2012, 18: 409 – 416.

作者：**Haney Mallemat, John Greenwood**

危重病

86. Ventilator-Associated Pneumonia?

1. Background

1) Definition: Pneumonia that occurs within 48 - 72 hours of ventilation.

2) Responsible for 50% ICU infections.

3) 1 in 5 patients who are intubated develop pneumonia!

4) Increases LOS, days intubated, and mortality.

2. Why does it happen?

1) ETT itself takes away host defenses.

2) Cuff inflation traps secretions, causes colonization, and bacteria transcend down into the lungs.

3) Oral flora changes in first 12 - 24 hours.

3. How can we prevent it?

1) Cheap

(1) Cleaning the mouth with chlorhexidine immediately after intubation, and every 12 hours, decreases the rate of tube colonization and incidence of VAP.

(2) Keep cuff pressure between 20 - 30 cm H_2O—need to check every 4 hours .

(3) Use H_2 blockers or sucralfate instead of PPIs.

(4) Elevate the HOB 30 - 45° (higher is better if no contraindications).

2) Expensive (none have been shown to improve outcomes)

(1) ETT w/subglottic suctioning apparatus.

(2) Antibiotic or silver-coated ETT.

4. BOTTOM LINE

1) VAP kills, and we have the power to prevent it!

2) Create a bundle that incorporates preventative measures, so that they happen every time.

Author: Haney Mallemat, MD

86. 呼吸机相关肺炎(VAP)

1. 背景
1)定义：在呼吸机使用48~72 h内出现的肺炎。

2)在ICU感染中占50%。

3)每5位气管插管的患者中会有1位发生肺炎。

4)增加住院时间、插管天数和死亡率。

2. 发生原因
1)气管导管本身解除了正常的宿主防御机制；

2)充气的气囊会使分泌物和细菌滞留，造成细菌下行到肺；

3)口腔菌群会在最初的12~24 h内改变。

3. 预防措施
1)便宜的方法

(1)插管后立刻用氯已定清洁口腔，然后每12 h一次，可减低导管内细菌滞留和VAP的发生率；

(2)保持气囊压力20~30 cmH_2O(要每4 h检查一次)；

(3)用H_2阻滞药或硫糖铝，不要用质子泵抑制药(PPIs)；

(4)将床头抬高30°~45°(如无禁忌证可再高一些)。

2)较昂贵的方法(均没有明确的改善预后的效果)

(1)带有声门下抽吸装置的气管导管；

(2)抗生素或镀银的气管导管。

4. 要点
1)VAP是致命的，但是我们可以预防它！

2)建立一个有效的预防方案，每一次都会严格遵循。

参考文献：

Grap MJ, Munro CL, Unoki T, et al. Ventilator-associated Pneumonia: The Potential Critical Role of Emergency Medicine in Prevention. JEM. 2012, 42(3): 353-362.

Kollef MH. Ventilator-associated complications, including infection-related complications. Crit Care Clin, 2013, 29: 33-50

作者：**Haney Mallemat, MD**

危重病

87. Anaphylaxis

1. Diagnosis involves 3 criteria, only have to meet one:

1) Sudden onset of illness (minutes-hours) w/involvement of skin/mucosa & either the upper/lower respiratory or cardiovascular systems.

2) 2 or more of the following that occur suddenly after exposure to a known or likely antigen: 1. Skin or mucosa involvement, 2. Respiratory symptoms, 3. Cardiovascular symptoms, 4. GI symptoms.

3) Hypotension (SBP <90 mmHg or 30% decrease from baseline).

2. Treatment

1) Epinephrine is the key! * * * Cardiac arrest can occur in 5 minutes of envenomation, 15 minutes of drug exposure, 30 minutes of food * * * Give IM immediately (mid-anterolateral thigh); 0.1 mg/kg (up to 0.3 mg); Repeat in 5 minutes if doesn't work (1:1000 epinephrine); Low-dose continuous infusion if no response to 2 IM injections (1:10, 000 at 1 – 10 mcg/min).

2) IVF: 1/3 of patient's effective circulating volume can be extravasated within 10 – 15 minutes!!! Give 10 mL/kg fluids in first 5 – 10 minutes.

3) H1-blockers (diphenhydramine, cetirizine): No high quality studies prove usefulness in anaphylaxis; Take 1 – 2 hours to work; Decrease itching, urticaria, and nasal symptoms; Older and newer agents work equally well.

4) H2-blockers (ranitidine): No high quality studies prove usefulness in anaphylaxis; Enhance the relief of urticaria & tachycardia; Ranitidine 50 mg IV or 1mg/kg over 15 minutes.

5) Glucocorticoids (methylprednisolone, prednisone): No high quality studies prove usefulness in anaphylaxis; Take hours to work; In theory, may reduce risk of biphasic symptoms.

6) Glucagon: For patients who have anaphylaxis and are on a beta-blocker, should consider giving glucagon because epinephrine may not work; 5 – 10mg.

7) Patients who are discharged MUST receive epinephrine pen (or Rx)

3. Disposition

1) Remember that biphasic reactions can happen up to 3 days later -and occur in 1

out of 4 patients!

2) Have to look at each individual patient; 6 – 8 hours has no good eviden.

4. BOTTOM LINE

1) Anaphylaxis is a fairly broad diagnosis.

2) Don't be afraid of epinephrine! It's the only drug that will save a life in anaphy-laxis.

3) Make sure there's an algorithm/care set for anaphylaxis for your ED.

Authors: Mike Winters, MD & Ellen Lemkin, MD

危
重
病

87.（严重）过敏性反应

1.诊断：包括3个标准，至少要符合其中之一：

1）突然发病（几分钟至几小时内），涉及皮肤、黏膜、上下呼吸道或心血管系统。

2）在接触已知或可疑过敏原后突然出现2个或2个以上的如下症状：①皮肤或黏膜症状；②呼吸症状；③心血管症状；④胃肠道症状。

3）低血压（收缩压＜90 mmHg或比基础血压降低30%）。

2.治疗

1）肾上腺素是关键！心脏骤停可在毒蛇咬伤5 min，药物接触15 min，食物接触30 min内出现。应立即肌内注射肾上腺素（股四头肌外侧）0.1 mg/kg（1 : 1 000稀释，最大剂量0.3 mg），如无效5分钟后可重复，如用两次肌注都无反应，可用低剂量（1 ~ 10 μg/ min）持续注射（1 : 10 000）。

2）静脉输液：1/3患者的有效循环容积会在10 ~ 15 min内渗到血管外！！！因此在前5 ~ 10 min内要给予10 mL/kg的液体。

3）H1拮抗药（苯海拉明、西替利嗪）：没有高质量的研究证实它们在严重过敏反应中的效用；1 ~ 2 h后起效；可减轻痒、荨麻疹和鼻部症状；新旧药物药效相当。

4）H2拮抗药（雷尼替丁）；没有高质量的研究证实它们在严重过敏反应中的效用；加速荨麻疹和心动过速的缓解；雷尼替丁50 mg静脉注射或1 mg/kg在15 min内滴注。

5）糖皮质激素（甲基强的松龙，强的松）：没有高质量的研究证实它们在严重过敏反应中的效用；数小时后起效；理论上来说，可能会防止症状的二次反复。

6）胰高血糖素：对于服用β受体阻滞药的过敏患者，因肾上腺素可能无效，可考虑使用高血糖素（5 ~ 10 mg）。

7）出院的患者一定要带肾上腺素自注笔（或处方）。

3.出院处理

1）记住1/4患者会出现二次反复，甚至在3 d以后发生！

2）因人而异，若没有证据支持只观察6 ~ 8 h就可以了。

4.要点

1）严重过敏反应是一个相当广的诊断。

2)不要畏惧肾上腺素！它是唯一能够在严重过敏反应时拯救生命的药物。

3)确保在你们科里建立一个治疗严重过敏反应的方案。

参考文献:

Simmons FER，Ardusso LRF，Bilo MB et al. 2012 update：World Allergy Organization guidelines for the assessment and management of anaphylaxs. Current Opinion in Allergy & Clinical Immunology，2012，12(4)：389 – 399.

作者：**Mike Winters，MD & Ellen Lemkin，MD**

危
重
病

88. Cardiorenal Syndrome?

1. Cardiorenal syndrome (CRS) type 1 is the development of acute kidney injury (AKI) in the patient with acute cardiac illness, most commonly acute decompensated heart failure (ADHF).

2. Multiple pathophysiological mechanisms result in CRS characterized by a rise in serum creatinine, oliguria, diuretic resistance, and worsening ADHF.

3. There are a host of predisposing factors that create baseline risk for CRS (DM, HTN, OSA).

4. The final common pathway often results in bidirectional organ injury, drug resistance, and death.

5. The combination of worsening renal function, volume overload, and diuretic refractoriness makes the management of CRS challenging.

6. Current therapies although often ineffective include aggressive diuresis and positive inotropes.

Author: Semhar Tewelde

88. 心肾综合征

1. 心肾综合征(CRS)1型是急性心脏疾病患者出现了急性肾损伤(AKI)，最常见的是急性失代偿性心力衰竭(ADHF)。

2. 多种病理生理机制导致了 CRS 的发生，其主要表现为血肌酐上升、少尿、利尿药抵抗及 ADHF 恶化。

3. 诱发 CRS 的基础危险因素有很多(糖尿病、高血压、阻塞性睡眠呼吸暂停综合征)。

4. 最后共同通路常常导致双向脏器损伤，耐药和死亡。

5. 肾功能恶化、容量超负荷、利尿药无效的同时存在，使 CRS 的处理更具有挑战性。

6. 虽然效果不理想，目前的治疗方法仍包括积极利尿和正性肌力药物的使用。

参考文献：

Ronco C, et al. Cardiorenal Syndrome Type I: Pathophysiological Crosstalk Leading to Combined Heart and Kidney Dysfunction in the Setting of Acutely Decompensated Heart Failure. JACC, 2012, 60 (12)

作者：**Semhar Tewelde**

危重病

89. Monitoring Hyperosmolar Therapy in Neurocritical Care?

1. Hyperosmolar therapy (mannitol or hypertonic saline) is commonly used in the treatment of neurocritical care paitents with elevated ICP.

2. When administering mannitol, guidelines recommend monitoring serum sodium and serum osmolarity. Though targets remain controversial, most strive for a serum sodium of 150 – 160 mEq/L and a serum osmolarity between 300 – 320 mOsm/L.

3. Unfortunately, serum osmolarity is a poor method to monitor mannitol therapy.

4. Instead of serum osmolarity, follow the osmolar gap. It is more representative of serum mannitol levels and clearance. If the osmolar gap falls to normal, the patient has cleared mannitol and may be redosed if clinically indicated.

Author: Michael Winters

89. 神经危重患者高渗治疗的监测

1. 高渗疗法(甘露醇或高渗盐水)是治疗伴有颅内压增高的神经外科危重患者的常用手段。

2. 当使用甘露醇时,指南建议监测血清钠和血渗透压。虽然对控制目标仍然有争议,许多人都用钠为 150～160 mEq/L,血清渗压 300～320 mOsm/L 作为控制目标。

3. 不幸的是,血清渗透压并不是监测甘露醇治疗的有效指标。

4. 除血清渗透压外,还要监测渗透间隙。它更能反映血清中的甘露醇水平和清除情况。如果渗透间隙下降至正常,说明患者体内甘露醇已被清除,如临床需要可以再补充甘露醇。

参考文献:

Hinson HE, Stein D, Sheth KN. Hypertonic Saline and Mannitol in Critical Care Neurology. J Intensive Care Med, 2013, 28: 3－11.

作者: **Michael Winters**

危
重
病

90. The Macklin Effect

1. Pneumomediastinum may be caused by many things:

1) Esophageal perforation (e. g. , complication from EGD).

2) Tracheal/Bronchial injury (e. g. , trauma, complication of bronchoscopy, etc.).

3) Abdominal viscus perforation with translocation of air across the diaphragmatic hiatus.

4) Air may reach mediastinum along the fascial planes of the neck.

5) Alveolar rupture, also known as the 'Macklin Effect'

2. The 'Macklin Effect' is typically a self-limiting condition leading to spontaneous pneumomediastinum and massive subcutaneous emphysema after the following:

1) Alveolar rupture from increased alveolar pressure (e. g. , asthma, blunt trauma, positive pressure ventilation, etc.).

2) Air released from alveoli dissects along broncho-vascular sheaths and enters mediastinum.

3) Air may subsequently track elsewhere (e. g. , cervical subcutaneous tissues, face, epidural space, peritoneum, etc.).

3. Pneumomediastinum secondary to the Macklin effect frequently leads to an extensive workup to search for other causes of mediastinal air. Although, no consensus exists regarding the appropriate workup, the patient's history should guide the workup to avoid unnecessary imaging, needless dietary restriction, unjustified antibiotic administration, and prolonged hospitalization.

4. Treatment of spontaneous pneumomediastinum includes:

1) Supplemental oxygen and observation for airway obstruction secondary to air expansion within the neck.

2) Avoiding positive airway pressure, if possible.

3) Avoiding routine chest tubes (unless significant pneumothorax is present).

4) Administering prophylactic antibiotics are typically unnecessary.

5) Ordering imaging as needed.

Author: Haney Mallemat

90. Macklin(麦克林)效应

1. 纵隔气肿可能由很多因素造成：

1）食管穿孔（如 EGD 的并发症）；

2）气管/支气管损伤（如外伤、支气管镜检查并发症等）；

3）腹部空腔脏器穿孔，气体通过膈肌裂孔进入纵隔；

4）气体可能沿颈部筋膜到达纵隔；

5）肺泡破裂，又称为"Macklin(麦克林)效应"。

2. "麦克林效应"通常是一个自限性过程，可导致自发性纵隔气肿和大面积皮下气肿，可在下列情况下发生：

1）肺泡内压增高导致肺泡破裂（如哮喘、钝器创伤、正压通气等）；

2）从肺泡释放的气体沿支气管血管鞘进入纵隔；

3）随后气体可能移行到其他地方（例如，颈部皮下组织、面部、硬膜外腔、腹膜等）。

3. 由麦克林效应产生的纵隔气肿往往会受到积极全面的评估，以寻找其他导致纵隔气肿的原因。虽然对于应做哪些合理的检查缺乏共识，然而患者的病史将有助于指导评估，以避免不必要的影像学检查、不必要的饮食限制、不合理的抗生素应用及延长住院时间。

4. 自发性纵隔气肿的治疗包括：

1）吸氧和观察由颈部气体膨胀导致的气道梗阻；

2）如果可能的话，避免气道正压通气；

3）避免常规放置胸导管（除非有严重的气胸）；

4）通常不需要预防性使用抗生素；

5）做必要的影像学检查。

作者：Haney Mallemat

危重病

201

91. Rhabdomyolysis in the Critically Ⅲ

1. Rhabdomyolysis can be disastrous in the critically ill patient, resulting in metabolic acidosis, life-threatening hyperkalemia, acute kidney injury, and acute renal failure (ARF). In fact, mortality can be as high as 60% for those that develop ARF secondary to rhabdomyolysis.

2. Although creatine kinase (CK) is a sensitive marker of muscle injury and used for diagnosis, it is actually the presence of myoglobinuria that results in ARF.

3. Current guidelines recommend treatment when the CK level is >5, 000 U/L.

4. The mainstay of treatment remains aggressive fluid resuscitation with crystalloids.

5. The administration of bicarbonate to alkalinize the urine, diuretics to increase urine output, and osmotic agents (mannitol) to augment urine output remain controversial and are not supported by current literature.

Author: Michael Winters

91. 危重患者中的横纹肌溶解症

1. 横纹肌溶解症对危重患者而言可能是灾难性的，导致代谢性酸中毒、危及生命的高钾血症、急性肾损伤和急性肾衰竭（ARF）。实际上，横纹肌溶解症导致的 ARF 死亡率可高达 60%。

2. 虽然肌酸激酶（CK）是肌肉损伤的敏感标志，可用于诊断，但实际上是肌红蛋白尿导致了 ARF。

3. 目前的指南建议 CK > 5 000 U/L 时要进行治疗。

4. 主要的治疗措施仍然是用晶体液积极进行液体复苏。

5. 使用碳酸氢钠碱化尿液，利尿剂及渗透剂（甘露醇）增加尿量的方法仍然存有争议，目前尚无文献支持。

参考文献：

Shapiro ML, Baldea A, Luchette FA. Rhabdomyolysis in the Intensive Care Unit. J Intensive Care Med, 2012, 27: 335 – 342.

作者：**Michael Winters**

危
重
病

92. NMBA Pearls in seriously ill patients

1. NMBAs are used in critically ill patients for RSI, patient-ventilator asynchrony, reducing intra-abdominal pressure, reducing intracranial pressure, and preventing shivering during therapeutic hypothermia.

2. There are a number of alterations in critical illness that affect the action of NMBAs

1) Electrolyte abnormalities.

2) Hypercalcemia: decreases duration of blockade.

3) Hypermagnesemia: prolongs duration of blockade.

4) Acidosis: can enhance effect of nondepolarizing agents.

5) Hepatic dysfunction: prolongs effects of vecuronium and rocuronium.

6) In addition, there are a number of medications that may interact with NMBAs

(1) Increased resistance: phenytoin and carbamazepine.

(2) Prolongs effect: clindamycin and vancomycin.

3. Key complications of NMBAs in the critically ill include:

1) ICU-aquired weakness (controversial).

2) DVT: NMBAs are one of the strongest predictors for ICU-related DVT.

3) Corneal abrasions: prevalence up to 60%.

Author: Michael Winters

92. 神经肌肉阻断剂(NMBA) 在危重患者中的应用

1. NMBA 在危重患者中主要用于 RSI、患者与呼吸机不同步、降低腹内压、降低颅内压及防止低温治疗过程中的颤抖。

2. 有许多严重疾病会影响 NMBAs 的作用

1)电解质紊乱；

2)高钙血症：缩短阻滞时间；

3)高镁血症：延长阻滞时间；

4)酸中毒：可增强非去极化剂的效应；

5)肝功能障碍：延长维库溴铵和罗库溴铵的效应；

6)此外，也有一些药物可能会影响 NMBAs：

(1)增加耐受力：苯妥英钠和卡马西平；

(2)延长作用时间：克林霉素和万古霉素。

3. 危重患者使用 NMBA 主要并发症包括：

1)ICU 获得性衰弱(有争议)；

2)DVT：NMBA 是与 ICU 相关 DVT 的最强预测因子；

3)角膜擦伤：患病率高达 60% 。

参考文献：

Greenberg SB, et al. The use of neuromuscular blocking agents in the ICU：Where are we know? Crit Care Med, 2013, 41：1332 − 1344.

危重病

93. How to warm your frozen patient

1. A 50yo man found down in the snow was brought into our ER last week in cardiac arrest with a bladder temperature of 21℃. Let's warm him up!

2. Passive external warming (good for mild hypothermia > 34℃): remove all wet clothing, use warm blankets.

3. Active external rewarming (Used for temp between 30 – 34℃): Radiant heat, electric blankets, Bair-Hugger. Disadvantages: "core temperature after drop" theory: drop in core temp because of peripheral vasodilatation. Therefore, focus on warming the chest and torso area. May not occur with certain warming techniques.

4. Active core rewarming (< 30℃, above techniques and several other options):

1) Heated humidified oxygen via mechanical ventilation at 42 – 46℃.

2) IV normal saline warmed to 41 – 43℃.

3) Cardio-pulmonary bypass: 1 – 2℃ increase every 5 minutes.

4) ECMO (best option in cardiac arrest): Up to 4 – 6℃/hr. VV or VA ECMO. Provides Cardio-pulmonary support. Can continue CPR while placing a cannula.

5) CVVH less costly, more available, 1 – 4℃/hr. Case reports only.

6) Artic Sun; external rewarming pads: used in hypothermia protocols. Easy to use. Case reports only.

5. Other methods (use if other methods are unavailable):

1) Pleural irrigation: one chest tube in the mid-clavicular line w saline at 42℃ and another chest tube in the post-axillary line and connected to a pleurovac.

2) Peritoneal lavage: 8 Frcatheter into the peritoneum using a standard paracentesis method. Use 40 – 45℃ dialysate.

3) Gastric, bladder, colonic irrigations.

6. We were able to get ROSC with CPR and ACLS and then used Artic Sun to rewarm successfully.

7. Other tips/tricks:

1) Continue CPR while rewarming (This is debatable: monitor ECG for new rhythms).

2) How warm is "warm and dead"? Probably around 32℃.

3) How fast to rewarm? Would warm quickly in cardiac arrest and then $1-2\,^{\circ}\text{C}/\text{hr}$ thereafter. (No good evidence here)

4) Arrhythmias corrected by rewarming (bradycardiaetc); no need for pacing.

5) Up to three defibrillations for V. fib/V. tach; hold if no benefit.

6) Can give epinephrine per ACLS protocol but would be cautious with further dosing.

7) Pressors: can use epinephrine drip cautiously for hypotension.

8) Cisatracurium for paralysis w/sedation to prevent shivering.

9) Rule out hypoglycemia, adrenal insufficiency, hypothyroidism, sepsis if patient does not rewarm as expected!

10) Avoid IJ lines or irritating the myocardium with a guidewire.

11) $K^+ > 12$ mmol/L: consider termination of CPR.

Author: Feras Khan

危
重
病

93. 如何对冰冻患者进行复温

1. 一星期前一位 50 岁的男性被发现躺在雪里。当他被送到急诊科时,他的心脏已停跳,膀胱温度为 21℃。下面就让我们给他复温吧!

2. 被动外部加温(适合轻度低温 > 34℃):脱掉所有的湿衣服,用温暖的毛毯。

3. 主动外部加温(30 ~ 34℃):辐射热、电热毯、Bair-Hugger 加热器。缺点:"中心温度下降"理论即由于外周血管扩张而导致中心温度下降。因此应主要对胸部和躯干区域加温。可能有些加温方法不会出现这种现象。

4. 主动中心加温(<30℃,上述技术和其他几项):

1)用加热(42 ~ 46℃)和湿化的氧气进行机械通气。

2)用加热到 41 ~ 43℃ 的生理盐水行静脉输液。

3)心肺体外循环:每 5 min 增加 1 ~ 2℃。

4)ECMO(心脏骤停时的最佳选择):升温可达 4 ~ 6℃/h。可用 VV 或 VA EC-MO 治疗。提供心肺支持。放置导管时可以继续心肺复苏。

5)CVVH:成本更低,更容易获得,升温 1 ~ 4℃/h。但只有个案报告。

6)北极太阳;外部复温垫,用于低温方案。易于使用。只有个案报告。

5. 其他方法(如果上述方法都无法使用时):

1)胸腔灌洗:从锁骨中线的胸导管灌入 42℃生理盐水,将另一个在腋后线的胸腔引流管连接到闭式引流器。

2)腹腔冲洗:使用标准腹腔穿刺术将 8F 导管插入腹腔。用 40 ~ 45℃ 的透析液冲洗。

3)胃、膀胱、结肠灌洗

6. 我们通过 CPR 和 ACLS 方案取得了 ROSC,然后用北极太阳来成功地复温。

7. 其他提示/技巧:

1)在复温的同时继续心肺复苏(这是值得商榷的:心电图监测心律改变)。

2)什么样的温度可以说"温暖死亡"? 约 32℃。

3)复温速度为多大? 心脏骤停时要快速复温,然后 1 ~ 2℃/h(关于这点缺乏很好的循证依据)。

4)复温可纠正心律失常 (心动过缓等)且无需起搏。

5)对室颤/室速最多除颤 3 次,如无效,不要再除颤。

6)可以按 ACLS 方案给肾上腺素，但再给药要谨慎。

7)升压药：如血压低可小心滴注肾上腺素。

8)防止发抖可用镇静药顺式阿曲库铵进行麻痹。

9)如果患者不能预期复温，要排除低血糖、肾上腺皮质功能不全、甲状腺功能减退症、脓毒症！

10)避免放置颈内静脉导管或用导丝刺激心肌。

11)K$^+$ >12 mmol/L 时要考虑终止心肺复苏。

参考文献：

nejm_hypothermia2012. pdf（581 kb）

作者：**Feras Khan**

危
重
病

94. Hypothermia

1. Lidocaine is generally ineffective in preventing ventricular arrhythmias, as is cardiac pacing or atropine to increase the heart rate.

2. Should the patient fully arrest be prepared to perform CPR for a long time. If your ED does not have a automatic CPR device consider calling your local fire department or ambulance service as they might have one that can be loaned to your department.

3. Warm fluids, heated blankets and heat lamps will typically increase a patients temperature about 1°C an hour.

4. Gastric lavage, peritoneal lavage and heated IV fluids can warm as much as 3' an hour.

5. To rewarm quickly as high as 18°C an hour requires cardiac bypass or thoracic lavage.

6. Finally, remember to monitor the patient closely when you first start rewarming as this can induce cardiac arrest. This is thought to occur as colder peripherial blood returns to the central circulation as peripherial veins and arteries dilated from the warm fluid.

Author: Michael Bond

94. 低温的急救

1. 利多卡因在预防室性心律失常时一般是无效的，就像心脏起搏或阿托品对心率增加没有帮助一样。

2. 如果患者处于心脏骤停，要准备进行长时间的心肺复苏。如果没有自动心脏按压设备，考虑向当地的消防队或救护服务公司求助，因为他们可能会有。

3. 温暖的液体、电热毯和热灯，通常会使患者温度每小时增加约1℃。

4. 洗胃、腹腔灌洗和加热的液体静脉输入可以使患者温度每小时增加约3℃。

5. 要以18℃/h的速度复温，需要体外循环或胸腔灌洗。

6. 最后，记住要密切监测患者，当患者开始复温时，可诱发心脏骤停。通常认为这是由于外周静脉和动脉因温暖液体而扩张造成的更冷的外周血返回到中央循环所致。

作者：Michael Bond

危重病

神经疾病
Neurology

95. 2013 Stroke Guidelines:
Revised and New Recommendations
(Part 1: Pre-Intervention)?

1. On January 31, 2013, the American Heart Association (AHA) and the American Stroke Association (ASA) released new recommendations for the early management of acute stroke, replacing the 2007 guidelines and subsequent 2009 update.

2. Prehospital Care

1) Patients should be transported to the closest certified primary or comprehensive stroke center or, when such an institution is not available, the closest facility offering emergency stroke care.

2) In some instances, this may involve air medical transport and hospital bypass.

3) Field personnel should notify the receiving facility that a potential stroke patient will be arriving to facilitate resource mobilization.

3. Stroke Center Designation/Quality Improvement

1) The section highlights the emergence of comprehensive stroke centers and their integration into regional systems of care.

2) Teleradiology is developing as a resource while data continue to support the use of telemedicine and quality improvement processes in stroke care.

4. Emergency Evaluation and Diagnosis

Fibrinolytic therapy should now not be delayed while awaiting laboratory test results other than a glucose determination.

5. Imaging: Symptoms Unresolved

Noncontrast CT or MRI can exclude hemorrhage and hypodensity involving more than one third of the middle cerebral artery territory prior to fibrinolytic therapy.

6. Imaging: Symptoms Resolved

MRI remains preferred over CT for imaging patients with suspected TIAs because it can provide insight into whether a stroke has occurred.

7. Supportive Care/Addressing Complications

1) Cardiac monitoring for at least 24 hours is recommended to screen for arrhythmias.

2) Hypovolemia should be corrected with IV saline.

3) Supplemental oxygen should be administered to achieve >94% saturation.

4) Blood glucose <60 mg/dL should be treated, ideally to normal, and hyperglycemia should be treated to a range of 140 – 180 mg/dL.

5) See our previous pearl (3 – 11 – 2013) for new recommendations for BP management. "Blood Pressure Management Updates from the 2013 Acute Ischemic Stroke Guideline"

Author: Feng Xiao, MD

神
经
疾
病

95. 2013 年脑卒中指南：修改部分和新的建议摘要（第一部分：介入治疗前）

1. 2013 年 1 月 31 日，美国心脏协会（AHA）和美国脑卒中协会（ASA）联合发表了对急性脑卒中早期处理的新指南，同时废弃了 2007 年的指南和 2009 年对其的更新。

2. 院前处理

1）应将患者转运到最近的被认证的初级或综合性脑卒中中心。如没有这样的机构，要送到能够提供紧急脑卒中处理的医院。

2）在某些情况下，可能需要空中医疗转运和绕过几个医院。

3）现场医务人员要通知接受医院可能有一个脑卒中的患者，以帮助医院及时调动资源。

3. 脑卒中中心的认证和质量改善

这一部分强调了建立高级脑卒中中心并与地区急救体系相融合的重要性。

远程放射学将成为一种资源，同时其资料支持发展远程医学和质量改善在脑卒中治疗中的作用。

4. 急诊评估和诊断

除明确血糖外，不要因为等待其他实验结果而拖延溶栓治疗。

5. 影像：症状没有完全改善

非增强 CT 或 MRI 能够在给予溶栓前排除出血或发现超过 1/3 的大脑中动脉区域的低密度灶。

6. 影像：症状完全改善

在怀疑有 TIA 时，MRI 要优于 CT，因为它能够帮助判断患者是否发生了脑卒中。

7. 支持疗法/注意并发症

1）心电监测至少要持续 24 小时，以发现心律失常。

2）静脉注射生理盐水以纠正低血容量。

3）给氧以保证血氧饱和度超过 94%。

4）血糖如低于 60 mg/dL，要进行纠正，争取达到正常；高血糖要纠正到 140～180 mg/dL 范围内。

5）参考我们在 2013 年 3 月 11 日发表的"2013 年急性缺血性脑梗死指南对血

压处理的更新"以了解对血压处理的新建议。

参考文献:

Edward C. Jauch, et al. Guidelines for the early management of patients with acute ischemic stroke: a guideline for healthcare professionals from the American Heart Association/American Stroke Association. Stroke, 2013, 44: 870 – 947.

作者: Feng Xiao, MD (肖锋)

神
经
疾
病

217

96. 2013 Stroke Guidelines:
Revised and New Recommendations
(Part 2: Interventions)

1. Intravenous Fibrinolysis

1) Eligible patients should receive rtPA therapy as soon as possible, ideally within 60 minutes of hospital arrival.

2) IV fibrinolysis can be considered in patients with rapidly improving symptoms, mild stroke deficits, major surgery within the past 3 months, and recent myocardial infarction.

3) The effectiveness of sonothrombolysis for treatment of patients with acute stroke is not well established.

4) rtPA is not recommended in patients taking direct thrombin inhibitors or direct factor Xa inhibitors unless tests including activated partial thromboplastin time, INR, platelet count, clotting time, thrombin time, or direct factor Xa activity are normal; or they haven't taken these agents for >2 days.

2. Endovascular Interventions

1) Select patients with MCA strokes of <6 hours duration who are not IV rtPA candidates can benefit from intra-arterial fibrinolysis.

2) Minimizing delays in administering intra-arterial fibrinolysis improves outcomes.

3) Stent retrievers are preferred to coil retrievers.

4) In patients with a large artery stroke who have not responded to IV fibrinolysis, intra-arterial fibrinolysis and mechanical thrombectomy are reasonable approaches.

5) Emergent intracranial angioplasty and/or shunting do not have proven usefulness, nor does the use of these approaches in the extracranial carotid or vertebral arteries in unselected patients.

Author: Feng Xiao, MD

美
国
急
诊
临
床
必
知
200
招

96. 2013 年脑卒中指南：修改部分和新的建议摘要 （第二部分：介入治疗）

1. 静脉溶栓

1）有适应证的患者应尽快接受 rtPA 治疗，最理想的是在到达医院后 60 min 内。

2）下列情况仍可以考虑静脉溶栓：症状很快改善，轻度缺血性脑卒中，过去的 3 个月内做过大手术和近期发生心肌梗死。

3）超声溶栓在治疗急性脑卒中中的效果还不清楚。

4）如患者正在使用直接凝血酶抑制药或 Xa 因子抑制剂，就不推荐使用 rtPA，除非下列检查正常或患者两天以上没有服用这些药：部分活性凝血酶原时间、INR、血小板计数、凝血时间、凝血酶时间或直接 Xa 因子活性。

2. 血管内介入治疗

1）对于发病 6 个小时内不适于静脉 rtPA 的大脑中动脉脑梗死的患者，可以考虑用动脉内溶栓。

2）尽快动脉内溶栓可以改善预后。

3）支架取栓要优于线圈取栓。

4）如患者大动脉脑梗死又对静脉溶栓无效，可以考虑用动脉内溶栓或机械取栓术。

5）紧急颅内血管扩张和/或分流没有明确的临床效果，它们在颅外颈动脉或椎动脉中的应用也一样未被证实有效。

参考文献：

Edward C. Jauch, et al. Guidelines for the early management of patients with acute ischemic stroke: a guideline for healthcare professionals from the American Heart Association/American Stroke Association. Stroke, 2013, 44: 870 - 947.

作者：**Feng Xiao, MD**（肖锋）

神经疾病

97. 2013 Stroke Guidelines:
Revised and New Recommendations
(Part 3: Post-intervention)

1. Anticoagulation

The usefulness of argatroban and other thrombin inhibitors in acute ischemic stroke is not well established.

2. Antiplatelet Agents

Aspirin remains the only antiplatelet agent for which data support use in acute stroke, although trials with other agents are in progress.

3. Volume Expansion, Vasodilators, and Induced Hypertension

Vasodilators are not recommended; Consider vasopressors with symptomatic hypotension; Efficacy of drug-induced hypertension and hemodilution by volume (i. e. , albumin) not well established.

4. Neuroprotection and Surgery

Hyperbaric oxygen is not recommended, except for air embolization; Continue statins; Transcranial near-infrared laser therapy and other neuroprotective drugs not recommended

5. Hospital Admission and Treatment

1)Nasogastric, nasoduodenal, or percutaneous endoscopic gastrostomy tube feeding should be used in patients unable to take liquids or solid food.

2) Nasogastric feeding is preferred to percutaneous endoscopy gastrostomy tube feeding until 2 – 3 weeks post-stroke in patients who cannot take oral liquid and food.

3)In patients in whom anticoagulation is contraindicated for DVT prophylaxis, consider external compression devices.

4) Routine nutritional supplements and prophylactic antibiotics have not been shown to be beneficial.

6. Treating Neurologic Complications

1)Aggressive medical treatment has been previously recommended in deteriorating patients with malignant edema due to a large cerebral infarction; however, the usefulness of this approach is not well established.

2)Decompressive surgical evacuation of a space-occupying cerebellar infarction can prevent and treat herniation and potential compression of the brain stem. Decompressive surgery is also effective for malignant cerebral edema.

3)In cases of stroke-induced acute hydrocephalus, a ventricular drain can be considred.

Author: Feng Xiao, MD

神
经
疾
病

97. 2013 年脑卒中指南：修改部分和新的建议摘要（第三部分：介入治疗后）

1. 抗凝治疗

阿加曲班及其他凝血酶抑制药对急性缺血性脑卒中的疗效还未被很好地证实。

2. 抗血小板药

阿司匹林仍是唯一的一个有证据支持在急性脑卒中使用的抗血小板药，其他的药物还在试验中。

3. 扩容、血管扩张药和诱导性高血压

不建议使用血管扩张药；如有症状性低血压可考虑升压药；药物诱发的高血压和容积性血液稀释（白蛋白）的效果还不明确。

4. 神经保护和手术

除非发生气体栓塞，否则不建议高压氧治疗；继续用他汀类药物；不建议用经颅近红外激光疗法和其他的神经保护药。

5. 住院治疗

1）如患者不能进液体或固体食物，要考虑鼻胃管，鼻十二指肠管或经皮内窥镜胃造瘘管。

2）鼻胃管对脑卒中后 2～3 周内不能从口进液体或固体的患者要优于经皮内窥镜胃造瘘管。

3）为防止 DVT 的发生，如不能用抗凝药，可考虑用体外压缩设备。

4）常规营养补充和预防性抗生素应用还未显示出益处。

6. 神经合并症的处理

1）虽然过去建议对由于大面积脑梗死造成的恶性脑水肿要进行积极药物治疗，但这些方法的效果还不清楚。

2）以减压为目的的小脑占位性梗死病灶的手术清除可以预防和治疗脑疝和对脑干的压迫。减压手术对恶性脑水肿也是有效的。

3）由脑卒中造成的急性脑积水的患者，可考虑行脑室引流。

参考文献:

Edward C. Jauch, et al. Guidelines for the early management of patients with acute ischemic stroke: a guideline for healthcare professionals from the American Heart Association/American Stroke Association. Stroke, 2013, 44: 870 – 947.

作者: **Feng Xiao, MD**（肖锋）

神经疾病

98. Blood Pressure Management Updates from the 2013 Acute Ischemic Stroke Guideline

The newest iteration of ' Guidelines for the Early Management of Patients with A-cute Ischemic Stroke' was recently published. Here are the key revisions specific to blood pressure management.

1. In patients with markedly elevated blood pressure who do not receive fibrinoly-sis, a reasonable goal is to lower blood pressure by 15% during the first 24 hours after onset of stroke. The level of blood pressure that would mandate such treatment is not known, but consensus exists that medications should be withheld unless the systolic blood pressure is >220 mmHg or the diastolic blood pressure is >120 mmHg.

2. No data are available to guide selection of medications for the lowering of blood pressure in the setting of acute ischemic stroke. Labetalol and/or nicardipine are listed as preferred, but other options can be used.

3. Restarting antihypertensive medications is reasonable after the first 24 hours for patients who have preexisting hypertension and are neurologically stable.

4. If administering rtPA, blood pressure needs to be <185/110 mmHg. That rec-ommendation didn't change.

Author: Bryan Hayes

美
国
急
诊
临
床
必
知
200
招

98. 2013 年急性缺血性脑梗死指南对血压处理的更新

最新理念的"急性缺血性脑卒中早期治疗的指南"刚刚发表，下面是几个有关血压控制的关键论点。

1. 对于血压明显增高但又不适合溶栓的患者，合理的目标是在发病24 h 内将血压降低15%。但什么水平的血压需要这样的处理还不清楚。专家一致公认的是，只要收缩压不高于 220 mmHg 或舒张压不高于 120 mmHg，就不要使用降压药。

2. 在急性缺血性脑卒中情况下如何选择降压药，还没有参考数据。拉贝洛尔和/或尼卡地平是首选的，但也可以有其他的选择。

3. 在第一个 24 h 后，对发病前患有高血压并且神经方面症状稳定的患者可以考虑恢复降压药的使用。

4. 如用 rtPA，血压需要控制在低于 185/110 mmHg。这方面的建议没有改变。

参考文献：

Jauch EC, et al. Guidelines for the early management of patients with acute ischemic stroke: a guideline for healthcare professionals from the American Heart Association/American Stroke Association. Stroke, 2013, Jan 31 [Epub ahead of print]. PMID 23370205.

作者：Bryan Hayes

神经疾病

225

99. tPA for Acute Ischemic Stroke Patients on Warfarin

1. IV alteplase (tPA) has many contraindications when administered for acute ischemic stroke. Among them is a history of warfarin use with INR $>1.7(0-3$ hours) or any history of warfarin use regardless of INR $(3-4.5$ hours).

2. A recent retrospective analysis of a major stroke registry compared the risk of symptomatic intracerebral hemorrhage (ICH) following tPA in patients on warfarin with an INR $<1.7(n=1,802)$ with patients not on warfarin therapy $(n=21,635)$.

3. After adjusting for differences in the two populations, the authors found no increased symptomatic ICH risk in patients with preadmission warfarin use $(5.7\%$ vs. 4.6%, $p=0.94)$.

4. Issue 1: Mean INR in study patients was only 1.22 (median 1.2). An INR of 1.2 represents very little actual anticoagulation.

5. Issue 2: In the small subgroup of patients with INR 1.5 to $1.7(n=269)$ there was a higher risk of ICH(7.8%), but did not reach statistical significance (it was significant in the unadjusted risk population).

6. Bottom line: Patients with INRs <1.5 may be ok to receive tPA. Patients with INRs 1.5 or greater need further study.

Author: Bryan Hayes

99. 服用华法林患者
急性缺血性脑卒中时 tPA 的应用

1. 静脉注射阿替普酶(tPA)在急性缺血性脑卒中使用中有很多禁忌证，其中包括服用华法林并且 INR > 1.7(0 ~ 3 h) 或只要服用华法林不管 INR 的值(3 ~ 4.5 h)。

2. 近期发表了一项大规模脑卒中回顾性分析报告，对接受 tPA 治疗脑出血症状服用华法林(INR < 1.7) 和不服用华法林患者之间出现的风险进行了比较。

3. 在对两组调查人群的差别进行校正后，作者发现华法林的使用并没有明显增加有症状的颅内出血的倾向(5.7% vs 4.6%，$p = 0.94$)。

4. 问题 1：研究组患者的 INR 只有 1.22(平均 1.2)。INR 1.2 只代表非常轻微的实际抗凝作用。

5. 问题 2：在 INR 1.5 ~ 1.7 亚患者组中，虽然没有明显统计学上的差别(在未校正前差异有统计学意义)，颅内出血率有增加(7.8%)。

6. 要点

INRs < 1.5 的患者接受 tPA 可能是没有问题的，但对于 INRs ≥ 1.5 的患者的安全性尚须进一步研究。

参考文献：

Xian Y, Liang L, Smith EE, et al. Risk of Intracranial Hemorrhage Among Patients With Acute Ischemic Stroke Receiving Warfarin and Treated with Intravenous Tissue Plasminogen Activator. JAMA, 2012, 307(24): 2600 – 2608.

作者：Bryan Hayes

神经疾病

100. tPA Use in Patients on New Oral Anticoagulants: Recommendations from the 2013 Ischemic Stroke Guidelines?

A new recommendation in the 2013 Ischemic Stroke Guidelines provides guidance on what to do in patients taking new oral anticoagulants who are deemed eligible for IV fibrinolysis. Here is what the guidelines say:

1. "The use of IV rtPA in patients taking direct thrombin inhibitors (dabigatran) or direct factor Xa inhibitors (rivaroxaban, apixaban) may be harmful and is not recommended unless sensitive laboratory tests such as APTT, INR, platelet count, and ECT, TT, or appropriate direct factor Xa activity assays are normal, or the patient has not received a dose of these agents for > 2 days (assuming normal renal metabolizing function)."

2. Additional points:

1) The most helpful lab tests are not widely available.

2) A detailed history is important, but not always obtainable.

3) Until further data are available, a history consistent with recent use of new oral anticoagulants generally precludes use of IV tPA.

Author: Bryan Hayes

美国急诊临床必知200招

100. 对于服用新型口服抗凝药的
患者如何使用 tPA：
2013 年缺血性脑卒中指南的建议

2013 年缺血性脑卒中治疗指南对适合使用静脉溶栓疗法但服用新的口服抗凝药的患者提供了一个新的建议。下面是指南在这一问题上的内容：

1."在使用直接凝血酶抑制药（达比加群）或直接 Xa 因子抑制药（利伐沙班、阿哌沙班）的患者中静脉应用 rtPA 可能是有害的，不建议使用。除非敏感的实验检查项目，如 APTT，INR，血小板计数，ECT，TT，或直接 Xa 因子活性测定正常，或患者在 2 天内没有服用过这些药物（假设患者肾脏代谢功能正常）。"

2.补充说明：

1）许多有意义的实验室检查并不普及。

2）详细的病史非常重要，但并不是任何时候都可以得到。

3）在有新的证据之前，近期服用过新的口服抗凝药的患者禁用静脉 tPA。

参考文献：

Jauch EC, et al. Guidelines for the early management of patients with acute ischemic stroke: a guideline for healthcare professionals from the American Heart Association/American Stroke Association. Stroke, 2013, 44(3): 870 - 947.

作者：**Bryan Hayes**

神
经
疾
病

101. What to tell patients who are eligible to receive tPA?

1. Remember that risk of intracranial hemorrhage is higher as severity of stroke goes up

2. Relatively young, healthy patients—smaller chance of intracranial hemorrhage ~4%

3. Older patients with comorbidities-increased chance of intracranial hemorrhage ~ 20%

4. More difficult to assess overall benefit of tPA

5. Improvement of function is a long process

6. Best to inform them function is not guaranteed nor is it necessarily to baseline but it is more likely with tPA

7. Ultimately, the decision is up to the patient so inform them adequately

8. Angioedema

1) An adverse reaction to tPA that is common but often not mentioned.

2) Occurs in 2% −5% of patients receiving tPA.

3) Usually not reversible.

4) Be prepared to intubate early should it occur.

5) Worth mentioning as a risk when doing consent for tPA.

Author: Michael Abraham, Bryan Hayes, and Sarah Dubbs

101. 要告诉 tPA 患者什么?

1. 要记住,颅内出血的风险将随脑卒中的严重程度的加重而增加。

2. 相对年轻和健康的患者——颅内出血的风险小,大约在 4%。

3. 年龄大且有并发症的患者——颅内出血的风险大,大约在 20%。

4. 很难评价 tPA 的准确效益。

5. 功能的恢复需要很长时间。

6. 最好要告诉患者,不能保证功能恢复或恢复到病前,但 tPA 的应用可增加功能恢复的可能性。

7. 最终的决定权在患者,因此一定要提供充分的信息。

8. 血管性水肿:

1)tPA 的不良反应之一,但经常被忽视;

2)在接受 tPA 的患者中发生率为 2% ~5%;

3)通常是不可逆的;

4)如出现血管性水肿,要准备早期气管插管;

5)在考虑 tPA 时,应当提及这一危险(血管性血肿)。

作者:Michael Abraham,Bryan Hayes,and Sarah Dubbs

神经疾病

102. tPA use in 4.5 – 6 hours of CVA

1. Background

1) Standard of care is to give tPA within 3 hours of symptom onset.

2) There is good data that suggests good outcomes in those even within 3 – 4.5 hour window.

3) These two articles look into if the window can be extended further to 6 hours.

2. Lancet article 1

1) Randomized control trial looking at around 3000 patients who had ischemic strokes within the 4.5 – 6 hour window since symptom onset.

2) 1500 patients received tPA and 1500 received a saline control.

3) Results found that tPA patients who survived 7 days up to 6 months had a comparable morbidity and mortality to those patients who did not receive tPA.

4) 245 died who received tPA vs. 300 died who did not receive tPA.

5) Before 7 days, 11% died who received tPA vs. 7% died who did not receive tPA

3. Lancet article 2

1) Wardlaw et al took 12 articles of patients who were given tPA within 6 hours, pooled their data, and looked at their outcomes through data analysis.

2) 7012 patients total.

3) Results showed chances of death increased within 7 days in the patients who got tPA (9% in those who received tPA vs. 6% in those who did not) and chance of symptomatic intracranial hemorrhage increased within 7 days (7.7% in those who received tPA vs. 1.8% in those who did not).

4) After 7 days, patients who received tPA were found to have higher benefit from a functional standpoint.

5) The number of deaths were similar between the two groups at 6 month follow up and the number with independent function was higher in patients who received tPA.

4. Bottom line:

No convincing evidence to suggest it is safe to give tPA for the 4.5 – 6 hour window.

Author: Michael Abraham, Bryan Hayes, and Sarah Dubbs

102. tPA 在脑卒中后 4.5~6 小时内的应用

1. 背景资料

1)脑卒中症状出现 3 h 内使用 tPA 是标准的治疗措施。

2)有研究显示在 3~4.5 h 内使用也可改善预后。

3)最近有两篇论文研究了是否可以将治疗窗延长到 6 h。

2. 柳叶刀文章 1：

1)随机对照试验，包括 3 000 名在发病后 4.5~6 h 内就诊的缺血性脑卒中的患者。

2)大约 1 500 人接受了 tPA，另外 1 500 人使用生理盐水作为对照。

3)结果显示接受 tPA 并存活 7 天到 6 个月患者的合并症和死亡率与没有接受 tPA 的患者相似。

4)tPA 组有 245 人死亡，对照组有 300 人死亡。

5)7 天内的死亡率 tPA 组为 11%，对照组为 7%。

3. 柳叶刀文章 2：

1)Wardlaw 等对 12 篇 6 h 内使用 tPA 的文章进行了总结，对他们的预后结果进行了分析。

2)一共有 7 012 个患者。

3)结果显示 tPA 增加了患者 7 d 内的死亡率(tPA 组为 9%，对照组为 6%)和有症状颅内出血的发生率(tPA 组为 7.7%，对照组为 1.8%)。

4)7 d 后，接受 tPA 治疗的患者在功能恢复方面要好于对照组。

5)在 6 个月的随访时间内，两组患者的死亡率相似，但独立功能恢复的人数在 tPA 组要高。

4. 要点

没有有力证据支持 tPA 在发病后 4.5~6 h 内的使用是安全的

参考文献：

IST – 3 Collaborative Group. The benefits and harms of intravenous thrombolysis with recombinant tissue plasminogen activator within 6 h of acute ischaemic stroke (the third international stroke trial [IST – 3]): a randomised controlled trial. The Lancet, 2012, 379 (9834): 2352 – 63, 23.

Wardlaw JM, Murray V, Berge E, et al. Recombinant tissue plasminogen activator for acute ischaemic stroke: an updated systematic review and meta-analysis. The Lancet, 2012, 379 (9834): 2364 – 2372.

作者：**Michael Abraham, Bryan Hayes, and Sarah Dubbs**

神经疾病

103. Infective endocarditis and tPA

1. Emergency Physicians face undeniable pressure to treat as many ischemic stroke patients with thrombolysis as possible, and as quickly as possible.

2. Current guidelines for IV tPA in acute ischemic stroke do not exclude patients with infective endocarditis.

3. However, infective endocarditis-related strokes are associated with a higher risk of hemorrhagic complications and recent experience suggests that IV tPA use may potentiate that risk and thrombolytic use in patients with IE-associated stroke is associated with very poor outcomes.

4. Cerebral complications are the most severe extracardiac complications of infective endocarditis, as well as the most frequent (occurring in 15 – 20% of patients). Ischemic and hemorrhagic stroke precede the diagnosis of infective endocarditis in 60% of patients.

5. Though diagnosis of IE in the acute stroke setting is difficult, clinical features (e. g. fever, a new murmur or worsening of a known murmur, hematuria) may raise concern for IE and should give the physician pause to consider the diagnosis.

Author: Feng Xiao

103. 感染性心内膜炎与 tPA

1. 由于许多缺血性脑卒中患者需要尽可能、越快越好地接受溶栓治疗，急诊医师面临着不可否认的压力。

2. 在新的静脉应用 tPA 治疗急性缺血性脑卒中的指南中，并没有将感染性心内膜炎的患者列为禁忌证。

3. 然而，感染性心内膜炎相关的脑卒中具有较高发生出血性并发症的风险，而近期临床经验表明静脉使用 tPA 可能会增加这一危险而使由感染性心内膜炎引起的脑卒中应用静脉溶栓预后很差。

4. 脑的并发症是感染性心内膜炎最严重且最常见的心外并发症（发生在 15% ～20% 的患者）。缺血伴出血性脑卒中发生在感染性心内膜炎诊断之前的占 60% 。

5. 虽然在急性脑卒中情况下诊断感染性心内膜炎是非常困难的，临床特征（如发烧、新杂音或一个已知的杂音的变化、血尿）可能会提高临床医生对感染性心内膜炎的警觉，并考虑这一诊断。

参考文献：

Bhuva P, et al. Neurocrit Care, 2010, 12：79 – 82.

Walker KA, et al. Neurohospitalist, 2012, 2：87 – 91.

Hoen B, et al. N Engl J Med, 2013, 368：1425 – 1433.

作者：**Feng Xiao**（肖锋）

神经疾病

104. Intensive BP Control
in Spontaneous Intracranial Hemorrhage

1. Managing the patient with hypertensive emergency in the setting of spontaneous intracerebral hemorrhage (ICH) is often a challenge. Current guidelines from the American Stroke Association are to target an SBP of between 160 – 180 mmHg with continuous or intermittent IV antihypertensives. Continuous infusions are recommended for patients with an initial SBP > 200 mmHg

2. An emerging concept is that rapid and aggressive BP control (target SBP of 140) may reduce hematoma formation, secondary edema, & improve outcomes.

3. Recently published, the INTERACT 2 trial (n = 2, 829) compared intensive BP control (target SBP < 140 within 1 hour) to standard therapy (target SBP < 180) found:

　　1) No difference in mortality (11.9% vs 12%, respectively).

　　2) Improved functional status (secondary outcome) with intensive BP control.

　　3) Intensive lowering of BP in patients with acute ICH appears safe.

4. A post-hoc analysis of the INTERACT 2 published just this month suggests that large fluctuations in SBP (> 14 mmHg) during the first 24 hours may increase risk of death & major disability at 90 days.

5. Bottom Line: INTERACT 2 was a large RCT but not a great study (keep on the look out for ATACHII). However, in patients with spontaneous ICH, consider early initiation of an antihypertensive drip (preferably nicardipine) in the ED to reduce blood pressure fluctuations early with a target SBP of 140 mmHg.

Author: John Greenwood

104. 自发性颅内出血时要加强血压控制

1. 处理高血压危象导致的自发性脑出血(ICH)患者往往是一个挑战。目前美国脑卒中协会的指南是通过持续或间歇静脉给降压药将收缩压控制在160~180 mmHg。患者初始收缩压 >200 mmHg 时要持续输注。

2. 新理念是快速和积极地控制血压(目标收缩压为 140 mmHg)可减少血肿形成,继发性水肿并改善预后。

3. 最近公布的 INTERACT2 试验($n=2,829$)将强化血压控制(1 h 内收缩压目标 <140 mmHg)和标准治疗(目标收缩压 <180 mmHg)进行比较,发现:

1)死亡率无明显差异(分别为 11.9% 和 12%);

2)强化血压控制改善了功能状态(次要结果);

3)积极降血压对急性脑出血患者是安全的。

4. 一项已发表的 INTERACT2 析因分析表明,在第一个 24 h 内收缩压的大幅度波动(>14 mmHg),可能会增加 90 d 内的死亡率和大部分生活不能自理的风险。

5. 要点

INTERACT2 是一项大型的随机对照试验,但并不是没有瑕疵的(可关注 AT-ACHII)。无论如何,对自发性脑出血患者,可考虑在急诊科尽快静脉使用降压药(尼卡地平最好),以减少血压波动并将收缩压控制在 140 mmHg 以内。

参考文献:

1. Morgenstern LB, Hemphill JC, Anderson C, et al. Guidelines for the management of spontaneous intracerebralhemorrhage: a guideline for healthcare professionals from the American HeartAssociation/American Stroke Association. Stroke, 2010, 41(9): 2108 – 2129.

2. Anderson CS, Heeley E, Huang Y, et al. Rapid blood-pressure lowering in patients with acute intracerebralhemorrhage. N Engl J Med, 2013, 368(25): 2355 – 2365.

3. Hill MD, Muir KW. INTERACT – 2: should blood pressure be aggressively lowered acutely after intracerebralhemorrhage?. Stroke, 2013, 44(10): 2951 – 2952.

4. Manning L, Hirakawa Y, Arima H, et al. Blood pressure variability and outcome after acuteintracerebralhaemorrhage: a post-hoc analysis of INTERACT2, a randomisedcontrolled trial. Lancet Neurol, 2014,

5. Qureshi AI, Palesch YY. Antihypertensive Treatment of Acute Cerebral Hemorrhage (ATACH) II: design, methods, and rationale. Neurocrit Care, 2011, 15(3): 559 – 576.

作者: John Greenwood

神经疾病

105. Status Epilepticus? Current Evaluation and Management Pearls

1. Although some controversy still remains, experts have recently defined SE as 5 minutes or more of continuous seizure activity. In part, this definition was adopted because most seizures that last longer than 5 minutes do not stop spontaneously.

2. Non-convulsive status epilepticus (NCSE) is a subset of SE defined as seizure activity seen on EEG without clinical findings associated with convulsive SE. Of particular relevance to the Emergency Physician, two distinct types of NCSE have been described:

1) the 'wandering confused' patient presenting to the ED; 2) the acutely ill patient with severely impaired mental status, with or without subtle motor movements.

3. Benzodiazepines are emergent initial therapy. For IV therapy, lorazepam is the preferred agent; midazolam is preferred for IM therapy. In one study IM midazolam was found to be at least as effective as IV lorazepam in prehospital patients with SE.

4. Following administration of benzodiazepines, urgent control antieplileptic drug (AED) therapy is required; the most common agents used are phenytoin/fosphenytoin, valproate sodium, and levetiracetam. At this stage, if attempts to control SE with bolus intermittent therapy fails, the patient is in refractory SE and continuous IV (cIV) AED is recommended.

5. However, the use of valproate sodium, levetiracetam, and phenytoin/fosphenytoin in intermittent boluses may also be considered if they have not previously been administered.

6. In actual practice, SE experts who care for adult patients choose cIV therapy for RSE, especially midazolam and propofol; and in children, there is a reluctance to choose propofol. Pentobarbital is chosen later in the therapy for all ages.

Author: Feng Xiao

105. 癫痫持续状态（目前的认识和处理要点）

1. 虽然仍有些争议，专家们最近定义癫痫持续状态（SE）为 5 min 或更长时间的持续惊厥。在某种程度上，采用这一定义，是因为大多数超过 5 min 的癫痫发作都不可能自行停止。

2. 非惊厥性癫痫持续状态（NCSE）是癫痫持续状态的亚型，是指患者有癫痫发作脑电图改变但无抽搐的临床表现。特别与急诊医师有关的两种不同的类型包括：1）到急诊科就诊的"迷茫徘徊"患者；2）急性危重患者伴严重精神状态改变，没有或只有轻微的抽搐。

3. 用苯二氮䓬类药物进行紧急的初始治疗。对于静脉注射治疗，劳拉西泮是首选药物；如肌肉注射可选用咪达唑仑。在一项对入院前癫痫持续状态患者的研究中发现，肌肉注射咪达唑仑与静脉注射劳拉西泮有同样的效果。

4. 在给苯二氮䓬类药物之后，必须要给抗癫痫药物（AED），最常见的 AED 为苯妥英钠/磷苯妥英钠、丙戊酸钠、左乙拉西坦。在这个阶段，如果用间歇静脉注射未能控制癫痫持续状态，患者属于难治性 SE，可考虑持续性静脉给予 AED。

5. 但是，如患者以前没有用过丙戊酸钠、左乙拉西坦、苯妥英/磷苯妥英，可考虑间歇静脉注射。

6. 在实际工作中，成人 SE 专家对顽固性 SE 通常选择持续 IV 治疗，尤其是咪达唑仑和丙泊酚；但对儿童来说，在选择丙泊酚时需谨慎。在治疗所有年龄患者的后续阶段，可考虑使用巴比妥。

参考文献：

Brophy GM, et al. Guidelines for the evaluation and management of status epilepticus. Neurocrit Care, 2012, 17: 3 – 23.

Shorvon S. What is nonconvulsive status epilepticus, and what are its subtypes? Epilepsia, 2007, 48(Suppl 8): 35 – 38.

Silbergleit R, et al. Intramuscular versus intravenous therapy for prehospital status epilepticus. N Engl J Med, 2012, 366: 591 – 600.

Riviello JJ Jr. et al. Treatment of status epilepticus: an international survey of experts. Neurocrit Care, 2013, 18: 193 – 200.

作者：**Feng Xiao**（肖锋）

神经疾病

106. Oral Phenytoin Loading

1. We often see seizure patients on phenytoin therapy who have subtherapeutic levels. Most patients do not require intravenous loading and can be adequately managed with oral treatment.

2. To estimate what dose to prescribe, use the following equation: [0.7 x IBW x (15 – current level)]. For example if a 70 kg patient has a level of 8 mcg/mL (mg/L), we would need ~400 mg loading dose to achieve a level of 15.

3. Phenytoin is known for its erratic absorption and propensity for causing GI upset with doses too high. The recommended strategy is to avoid administering more than 400 mg at one time and separate the doses by 2 hours. This would take three doses over 4 hours for a 1 gm load.

4. In the ED, an effective strategy for a 1 gm oral load is 500 mg now and 500 mg in 2 hours at discharge. Patients tolerate it well, it cuts down on ED length of stay, and still achieves therapeutic levels. Remember that an oral suspension formulation is also available.

Author: Bryan Hayes

106.苯妥英钠的口服负荷剂量

1. 我们经常会遇见一些服用苯妥英钠不足量的癫痫患者，大多数这样的患者可给予口服负荷量，并不需要静脉给药。

2. 估算所需口服剂量，可用下列公式：0.7 × 理想体质量 × (15 − 目前血浆浓度)。例如：苯妥英钠血浆浓度为 8 μg/mL(mL/L)的 70 kg 的患者，需要口服大约 400 mg 的负荷量以达到 15 μg/mL 的血浆浓度。

3. 苯妥英钠的消化道吸收是不稳定的，并且剂量太大可导致消化道症状。建议方法是避免一次剂量超过 400 mg，可隔 2 h 重复给药。这样 1 g 的口服负荷量可通过 3 次在 4 h 内完成。

4. 在急诊科，需要 1 g 口服负荷量的有效方法是立即给 500 mg，然后 2 小时后出院时再给 500 mg。患者对这样的方法耐受很好，在达到治疗浓度同时缩短了急诊科停留时间。记住，苯妥英钠也有口服的液体制剂。

作者：**Bryan Hayes**

神经疾病

107. Myasthenia Gravis

1. Work-up

1) Myasthenic crisis vs. cholinergic crisis (from medication OD).

2) History.

3) Myasthenic crisis: Generalized weakness, Worsening of ptosis.

4) Cholinergic crisis: SLUDGE.

5) Can do edrophonium test

1 – 2mg IV, expect improvement in 30 – 90 seconds, Can repeat with 3mg & then 5mg; if no improvement likely cholinergic crisis, Consider adding a medication to decrease secretions (ex. Glycopyrrolate), Must have atropine at the bedside, Adverse side effects: worsening of respiratory status.

6) Cold test: Place ice pack over eye-should have improvement in ptosis.

7) Triggers for crisis: Idiopathic worsening, Medication non-compliance, Infection (pneumonia most common), Medication interaction (particularly fluoroquinolones), Any physiologic stressor.

2. Who needs to be intubated?

1) ABG: Severe hypercarbia ($CO_2 > 50$).

2) NIF (negative inspiratory force), Surrogate marker of strength of chest wall musculature, < 20 cm H_2O: needs respiratory support.

3. Airway management

1) BiPap vs. intubation: BiPap may prevent ventilation, $CO_2 > 50$ on arrival predicts BiPap will fail, Reasonable to try if treatment (IVIG, etc. readily available).

2) RSI drugs: Consider sedation w/o paralysis, Non-depolarizing agents OK, but they'll last longer, Succinylcholine usually won't work, very unpredictable.

4. BOTTOM LINE

1) Patients in myasthenic crisis should be pan-cultured.

2) Intubate if $pCO_2 > 50$ or NIF < 20 cm H_2O.

3) Use rocuronium or vecuronium for RSI.

Authors: Mike Abraham, MD & Danya Khoujah

107. 重症肌无力

1. 诊断
1) 重症肌无力危象和胆碱能危象(药物过量)。
2) 病史。
3) 重症肌无力危象：全身无力，眼睑下垂加重。
4) 胆碱能危象：唾液增加，流泪，尿频，大便增多，瞳孔缩小，心率缓慢，支气管痉挛。
5) 腾喜龙试验：

静脉注射 1~2 mg，如在 30~90 秒内肌力好转为肌压力危象，可重复用 3 mg，然后 5 mg；如无改善，则可能是胆碱能危象，考虑加用抗胆碱药(格隆溴胺)，床旁需备阿托品；不良反应：呼吸困难加重。

6) 冷态试验：将冰块放在眼睛上，此时眼睑下垂应该改善。
7) 导致危象的原因：自发性的，用药不规律，感染(肺炎最常见)，药物反应(特别是氟喹诺酮)，生理应激。

2. 气管插管适应症
1) 血气：严重的高碳酸血症($PaCO_2 > 50$ mmHg)。
2) 负力吸气(NIF)是反映胸壁肌肉力量的指标，如 NIF < 20 cm H_2O，则需要呼吸支持。

3. 气道管理
1) BiPap 还是插管：BiPap 可避免插管，但患者到达时如 CO_2 超过 50 mmHg，意味着 BiPap 可能会失败，但在其他支持治疗(如丙种球蛋白等)就绪的情况下，可以尝试使用 BiPaP。
2) 气管内给药：可考虑单用镇静药，或合用肌肉松弛剂，可使用去极化肌肉松弛药，但它们持续时间较长；琥珀胆碱经常无效，非常难以预测。

4. 要点
1) 重症肌无力危象的患者都要做全部培养；
2) 如 $pCO_2 > 50$ mmHg 或 NIF < 20 cm H_2O，则需要插管；
3) 在插管时要用罗库溴铵或维库溴铵。

作者：Mike Abraham，MD & Danya Khoujah

神经疾病

243

108. Brain-Eating Amoeba!

1. General Information

1) Caused by the ameboflagellate Naegleria Fowleri.

2) Case fatality rate is estimated at 98%.

3) Commonly found in warm freshwater environments such as hot springs, lakes, natural mineral water, especially during hot summer months.

4) Incubation period 2 - 15 days.

2. Relevance to the EM Physician

1) Clinical presentation: resembling bacterial meningitis/encephalitis.

2) Final diagnostic confirmation is not achieved until trophozoites are isolated and identified from CSF or brain tissue.

3. Treatment: Amphotericin B

4. Bottom Line

History of travel to tropical areas or exposure to warm or under-chlorinated water during summer time should raise the suspicion for Naegleria Fowleri. The amoeba is not sensitive to the standard meningitis/encephalitis therapy and amphotericin B must be added to the treatment regimen.

Author: **Walid Hammad**

108. 侵蚀脑组织的阿米巴

1. 一般资料

1）由福氏耐格里阿米巴引起。

2）死亡率在98%以上。

3）常见于温暖的淡水环境，如温泉、湖泊、天然矿泉水，尤其是在炎热的夏季。

4）潜伏期2~15天。

2. 与急诊医师相关的内容

1）临床表现：类似细菌性脑膜炎/脑炎；

2）从脑脊液或脑组织分离和鉴定出滋养体才能确诊。

3. 治疗：两性霉素B。

4. 要点

有到热带地区旅游或夏季接触温水或未经氟气消毒的水的病史，应怀疑有福氏耐格里阿米巴感染。阿米巴对标准的脑膜炎/脑炎治疗不敏感，必需在治疗方案里加用两性霉素B。

参考文献：

Su MY, Lee MS, Shyu LY, Lin WC, Hsiao PC, Wang CP, Ji DD, Chen KM, Lai SC. A fatal case of Naegleria fowleri meningoencephalitis in Taiwan. Korean J Parasitol. 2013 Apr

Naegleria fowleri, Kelly Fero, ParaSite, February 2010 retrieved from

作者：**Walid Hammad**

神
经
疾
病

245

109. What should I MRI?

1. You have a patient with a spinal cord syndrome and you order the MRI. Have you ever had that conversation with radiology where you have to "choose" what part of the spine you want imaged?

2. The entire spine needs to be imaged!

3. The reason: False localizing sensory levels.

4. For example: The patient has a thoracic sensory level that is caused by a cervical lesion.

5. A study of 324 episodes of malignant spinal cord compression (MSCC) found that clinical signs were very unreliable indicators of the level of compression. Only 53 patients (16%) had a sensory level that was within 3 vertebral levels of the level of compression demonstrated on MRI.

6. Further, pain (both midline back pain and radicular pain) was also a poor predictor of the level of compression.

7. Finally, of the 187 patients who had plain radiographs at the level of compression at referral, 60 showed vertebral collapse suggesting cord compression, but only 39 of these predicted the correct level of compression (i. e. only 20% of all radiographs correctly identified the level of compression).

8. The authors note that frequently only the lumbar spine was XR at the time of clinical presentation, presumably due to false localizing signs and a low awareness on the part of clinicians that most MSCC occurs in the thoracic spine (68% in this series).

Author: Brian Corwell

109. 脊柱受损患者的核磁检查

1. 你有一个有脊髓受损表现的患者并准备要进行 MRI 检查。你是否与放射科有过交流,应该检查脊柱的哪个部位?

2. 应该照整个脊柱!

3. 理由:不能准确判断感觉异常水平。

4. 例如:患者胸椎感觉异常可能是由颈椎病变引起的。

5. 一个 324 例恶性脊髓压迫报告显示,在判断压迫水平时,临床体征是极为不可靠的。只有 53 个患者(16%)的异常感觉水平在 MRI 判断的压迫水平的 3 个锥体范围内。

6. 另外,疼痛(不管是后背正中痛或放射痛)也是一个非常差的判断压迫水平的指标。

7. 最后,在 187 个就诊时平片显示脊椎压缩水平的患者中,有 60 例的脊椎塌陷造成脊髓压迫,但只有 39 例与脊髓压迫水平相符(也就是说,只有 20% 的平片可以准确判断压迫的位置)。

8. 笔者认为,患者初诊时经常只对腰椎进行 X 线检查,可能是由于判断体征有误或临床医生对多数的恶性脊髓压迫发生在胸椎(此文献中占 68%)的概念认识不足。

参考文献:

Summers D, et al. Assessment of MSCC using MRI Br J Radiol 2001;74:977 – 8.

作者:Brian Corwell

神经疾病

呼吸系统急诊
Pulmonology

110. R. E. D. U. C. E. trial:
Is Less prednisone better?

1. COPD treatment guidelines (e. g. , GOLD) recommend 10 – 14 days of steroid therapy following a COPD exacerbation to prevent recurrences; the supporting data is weak.

2. A recent noninferiority trial compared patients with a severe COPD exacerbation who received either a 5 – day course (n = 156) or 14 – day course (n = 155) of prednisone 40 mg.

3. The results were:

1) No significant reduction in time until the next exacerbation (primary endpoint).

2) No significant difference in mortality, incidence of mechanical ventilation, FEV1, or dyspnea scores (secondary end-points).

4. What you need to know:

1) This was a non-inferiority trial, which has limitations.

2) All subjects received broad-spectrum antibiotics and an initial dose of IV steroid.

3) Surprisingly, there were no differences between groups with respect to steroid complications (e. g. , hyperglycemia, hypertension, etc.).

5. Bottom-line: 5 days of prednisone may be as effective as 14 – days for COPD exacerbations.

Author: Haney Mallemat

110. R. E. D. U. C. E.
研究结果：慢性阻塞性肺病的激素疗法

1. 慢性阻塞性肺病(COPD)的治疗指南(如 GOLD)建议在 COPD 恶化后使用激素治疗 10～14 天,可以防止复发,但支持这一观点的数据并不多。

2. 最近的一项非劣效性试验对 COPD 恶化后每天给予强的松 40 mg,连续 5 天($n = 156$)或 14 天($n = 155$)的患者进行了比较。

3. 结果如下:

1)到下一次发作的时间无明显缩短(主要指标);

2)死亡率、机械通气使用率、FEV1 或呼吸困难评分(次要指标)均无显著差异。

4. 你需要知道:

1)这是一个非劣效性试验,具有它的局限性;

2)所有实验者都接受了广谱抗生素和静脉注射初始剂量的激素;

3)令人惊讶的是,两组之间在激素并发症方面并无显著差异(例如高血糖、高血压等)。

5. 要点

对于慢性阻塞性肺病的急性发作,给予 5 天强的松治疗与 14 天同样有效。

参考文献:

Leuppi, JD, et al. Short-term vs conventional glucocorticoid therapy in acute exacerbations of chronic obstructive pulmonary disease: the REDUCE randomized clinical trial[J]. JAMA 2013 Jun 5; 309(21): 2223–2231.

作者: **Haney Mallemat**

呼吸系统急诊

111. Pulmonary Embolism:
7 Steps to Enlightenment!

1. Decreasing testing for pulmonary embolism (PE)

1) PERC rule (PE Rule-out Criteria)

(1) If a patient is PERC negative, there is a 0.3% chance of them having a PE.

(2) Unfortunately the test is not being used appropriately.

(3) If there is a low gestalt for PE, use PERC.

(4) If there is a higher risk of PE, PERC are not applicable.

2) Risk of radiation is high

1 radiation-induced malignancy for every 2000 pulmonary CT scans.

3) Risk of contrast-induced nephropathy (CIN).

1 case of CIN per 200 CT scans with IV contrast.

2. Seven step program

1) Step 1 – Accept that we cannot identify every PE.

2) Step 2 – Recognize that every strategy to detect PE does harm.

3) Step 3 – Risk stratification and reduce testing

(1) Low-risk patients should have PERC rules applied.

(2) Don't initiate diagnostic workups on people who you don't think have a PE.

4) Step 4 – Try watchful waiting

(1) Place patients in obs or have them return to ED or follow up with primary care physician in 24 hours to see if they are improved and then initiate testing.

(2) Document re-evaluation especially an actually counted respiratory rate.

5) Step 5 – Document the medical decision making

(1) Document why we don't think it is a PE and why it is not being worked up.

(2) Document the leg exam as well as the pulmonary exam.

(3) Show that you thought about if a DVT was present and there were no clinical signs of a DVT present.

6) Step 6 – Be less afraid of litigation

(1) Be thorough in the history and physical exam.

(2) Be nice to your patients.

7)Step 7 – Spread the word

(1)Teach our learners about whittling down the testing for PE.

(2)Teach them about the risks of excessive testing.

Author: Rob Rogers, MD

呼
吸
系
统
急
诊

111. 肺动脉栓塞：七步程序的启示

1. 减少诊断肺动脉栓塞(PE)的检查

1) 排除标准(PERC 原则)

(1) 如果一个患者的 PERC 阴性，只有 0.3% 的概率会有 PE。

(2) 不幸的是，这个标准没有被合理应用。

(3) 如临床诊断 PE 的可能性低，应采用 PERC。

(4) 如临床诊断 PE 的可能性高，不需进行 PERC。

2) 放射性危害是很大的

每 2 千个肺部 CT 扫描会造成一个由放射引起的恶性肿瘤。

3) 造影剂肾病(CIN)

每 200 个使用静脉造影剂的 CT 扫描会导致一个 CIN。

2. 七步程序

1) 第一步：承认我们不可能明确诊断每一个 PE。

2) 第二步：承认所有诊断 PE 的检查都是有害处的。

3) 第三步：危险因素分析及减少检查。

(1) 可能性低的患者应使用 PERC；

(2) 如你认为患者没有 PE，不要做诊断性的检查。

4) 第四步：密切观察患者。

(1) 观察患者或让患者在急诊室留观或家庭医生在 24 小时内随访，如无好转则进行诊断性检查。

(2) 对复诊患者要有记录，尤其是要对呼吸频率进行认真计数。

5) 第五步：记录你的决策根据。

(1) 记录为什么你认为患者没有 PE 和你没有做进一步检查的原因；

(2) 记录腿和肺部的检查；

(3) 证明你想到了患者有 DVT 或没有 DVT 的临床表现。

6) 第六步：不要太恐惧法律诉讼。

(1) 病史和体格检查一定要完整；

(2) 对患者一定要友好。

7) 第七步：做好宣传工作。

(1) 教育我们的学生要减少不必要的对 PE 的检查；

（2）让他们知道过度检查的危害。

参考文献：

Singh B, Parsaik AK, Agarwal D, et al. Diagnostic accuracy of pulmonary embolism rule-out-criteria: a systematic review and meta-analysis. Ann Emerg Med. 2012; 59: 517 – 520.

Green SM, Yealy DM. Right-sizing testing for pulmonary embolism: recognizing the risks of detecting any clot. Ann Emerg Med. 2012; 59: 524 – 526.

Vinson DR, Zehtabchi S, Yealy DM. Can selected patients with newly diagnosed pulmonary embolism be safely treated without hospitalization? A systematic review. Ann Emerg Med. 2012; 60: 651 – 662.

作者：**Rob Rogers, MD**

呼吸系统急诊

112. TRALI-Transfusion related lung injury

1. Background

1) Acute lung injury develops within 6 hours after transfusion of 1 or more units of blood or blood components.

2) Increased risk with greater number of transfusions.

3) Incidence is 1 in 4000.

2. Definition

1) Acute onset.

2) Hypoxemia ($PaO_2/FiO_2 < 300$ mm Hg).

3) Bilateral pulmonary opacities on chest x-ray.

4) Absence of left atrial hypertension.

3. Pathogenesis

Two-hit hypothesis: first hit is underlying patient factors causing adherence of neutrophils to the pulmonary endothelium; second hit is caused by mediators in the blood transfusion that activate the neutrophils and endothelial cells.

4. Differential

Can be confused or overlap with TACO or transfusion-associated volume/circulatory overload, which presents similarly but has evidence of increased BNP, CVP, pulmonary wedge pressure, and left sided heart pressures. Patients with TACO tend to improve with diuretic treatment.

5. Supportive tests

1) Echocardiogram.

2) BNP(tends to be low).

3) Transient leukopenia.

6. Treatment

1) Supportive care.

2) Lung protective ventilation strategies.

3) Fluid restrictive strategy.

4) Aspirin (shown to be helpful in animal studies).

5) Pre-washing of stored RBCs prior to transfusion.

6) Decrease the amount of transfusions!

Author: Feras Khan

112. TRALI – 与输血相关的急性肺损伤

1. 背景

1）急性肺损伤发生在输 1 个或多个单位的血液或血液成分后的 6 小时内。

2）随输血量增加，风险系数增大。

3）发病率为 1/4000。

2. 定义

1）起病急；

2）低氧血症（$PaO_2/FiO_2 < 300$ mmHg）；

3）胸片显示双侧肺实变影；

4）无左心房高压。

3. 发病机制

二次损伤假说：首先由造成疾病相关因素导致中性粒细胞黏附于肺血管内皮；然后由输血过程产生的炎症介质激活中性粒细胞和内皮细胞。

4. 鉴别诊断

可与输血相关的容量/循环超负荷（TACO）混淆或有重叠，TACO 表现虽类似，但有 BNP、CVP、肺动脉楔压、左心的压力增加的证据。TACO 患者通常在给予利尿药治疗后病情得以缓解。

5. 相关检查

1）超声心动图；

2）BNP 往往是低的；

3）短暂白细胞减少。

6. 治疗

1）支持治疗；

2）肺保护性通气措施；

3）限制液体量；

4）阿司匹林（在动物研究中证明是有助益）；

5）在输储存红细胞前进行冲洗；

6）减少输血量！

参考文献：

Lancet. 2013 Sep 14；382（9896）：984 – 94. doi：10. 1016/S0140 – 6736（12）62197 – 7. Epub 2013 May 1.

作者：**Feras Khan**

呼吸系统急诊

感染性疾病
Infectious Disease

113. Procalcitonin Algorithms to Guide Antibiotic Therapy in Upper Respiratory Infections (URIs)

1. Background:

1) Antibiotics are prescribed commonly for URIs including acute bronchitis and community acquired pneumonia.

2) Antibiotic prescriptions for non-bacterial causes of URIs lead to antibiotic overuse, which can lead to antibiotic resistance and risk of Clostridium difficile.

3) Procalcitonin is a biomarker for bacterial infections and is released in response to bacterial toxins during infections.

4) Several algorithms using procalcitonin have been developed to help guide antibiotic treatment of URIs based on blood levels and to aid discontinuing antibiotics when procalcitonin levels have returned to normal, leading to decreased use and length of antibiotic treatment courses.

2. Clinical Question:

Does measurement of procalcitonin lead to shorter antibiotic exposure without increasing mortality and treatment failure?

3. Meta-analysis:

14 trials; 2004 – 11; 4211 patients with a variety of URI severity and type including CAP and COPD exacerbations.

4. Inpatient and outpatient settings

1) Compared to regular antibiotic treatment without procalcitonin level guidance.

2) Primary outcomes: All cause mortality and treatment failure within 30 days.

5. Conclusions:

1) No increase in all-cause mortality using procalcitonin algorithms versus standard therapy in any clinical setting or type of URI (5.7% vs. 6.3%, respectively).

2) Treatment failure was LOWER for procalcitonin guided patients in the ED [OR 0.76 (95% CI, 0.61 –0.95)].

3) Lower antibiotic exposure due to lower prescription rate in COPD exacerbations and bronchitis.

6. Limitations：

1）Non-blinded to outcome assessment.

2）Adherence to algorithms was variable.

3）Immunosuppressed patients and children were excluded.

7. Bottom Line：

1）Another tool to help aid clinical decision making regarding antibiotic treatment

2）Test is around ＄25－30 and takes about 1 hour to run

3）Low levels may indicate a non-bacterial cause of infection.

Author：Feras Khan

感
染
性
疾
病

113. 降钙素原指导上呼吸道感染的抗生素治疗

1. 背景

1）在上呼吸道感染（URI），包括急性支气管炎和社区获得性肺炎（CAP），使用抗生素治疗是很常见的。

2）对非细菌性 URI 患者使用抗生素将导致抗生素的过度使用，增加抗生素耐药性和产生艰难梭状芽孢杆菌感染的风险。

3）降钙素原是细菌感染的生物指标，在感染过程中作为对细菌毒素的反应而被释放。

4）已有多种方案被提出，根据血中降钙素原水平指导抗生素在 URI 中的应用并提示当降钙素原恢复正常时可停止抗生素，进而减少了抗生素的应用并缩短了疗程。

2. 临床问题

在不增加死亡率和治疗失败条件下测量降钙素原可缩短抗生素的应用吗？

3. Meta 分析

14 个临床研究；2004－2011 年；4, 211 个严重程度和类型不同的 URI 患者，包括社区获得性肺炎和慢性阻塞性肺病急性发作。

4. 分别来自住院和门诊患者

1）与没有降钙素原水平指导的常规抗生素治疗进行对比。

2）主要指标：在 30 天内任何原因死亡和治疗失败。

5. 结论

1）与标准治疗相比，使用降钙素原无论在住院或门诊患者中还是各类型的 URI 中都没有增加全因死亡率（分别为 5.7% 和 6.3%）。

2）在急诊科使用降钙素原来指导患者的治疗失败率较低［OR = 0.76（95% CI, 0.61~0.95）］。

3）减少了慢性阻塞性肺病和支气管炎抗生素的使用率。

6. 文章缺点

1）对实验指标不盲；

2）对方案的执行情况有异；

3）免疫抑制患者和儿童被排除在外。

7. 要点：

1）可作为帮助临床决定是否需用抗生素的另一个指标；

2）检查大概需要 25～30 美元，一个小时出结果；

3）低水平可能意味着非细菌感染。

参考文献：

Philipp Schuetz；Matthias Briel；Beat Mueller. Clinical Outcomes Associated With Procalcitonin Algorithms to Guide Antibiotic Therapy in Respiratory Tract Infections［J］. JAMA. 2013；309（7）：717 －718. doi：10. 1001/jama. 2013. 697.

作者：**Feras Khan**

感
染
性
疾
病

114. Imported Pneumonia—what to worry about?

1. Case Presentation:

A 43 year old diabetic woman presents with dyspnea and a dry cough. Her vital signs are: BP 84/42, HR 135 RR 37 T 38.5. Lobar consolidation is seen on chest x-ray. She decompensates and is intubated, a central line is placed, and IV fluids are started. Her husband reports that they had just returned from a vacation in Thailand one week earlier.

2. Clinical Question:

Does the recent travel change your choice of empiric antibiotics?

3. Answer:

The patient should also be covered for melioidosis, and infection caused by Burkholderia pseudomallei.

4. Infection can occur via direct contact with, inhalation of, or ingestion of the bacteria.

5. B. pseudomallei is highly endemic in Thailand and Northern Australia, but melioidosis has been contracted in the Americas and other parts of Asia and Australia. (True epidemiology is unknown due to difficulties in culturing the bacteria)

6. Clinical presentation most frequently involves pulmonary infection, abscess formation, or bacteremia.

7. Labs that don't have experience with this bacteria have difficulty culturing it and it is often misidentified.

8. Treatment is 10 – 14 days of ceftazidime or a carbapenem.

9. After recovery, the patient requires TMP-SMX for 3 – 6 months for bacterial eradication.

10. Bottom Line:

Patients presenting with severe infections and recent travel to an endemic area should receive emperic antibiotics with ceftazidime or a carbapenem until another source is identified.

Author: Jenny Reifel Saltzberg

美国急诊临床必知200招

114. "进口"肺炎——需要警惕什么？

1. 病例简介

43 岁的女性糖尿病患者因呼吸困难和干咳就诊，她的生命体征：血压 84/42 mmHg，心率 135 次/分，呼吸 37 次/分，体温 38.5℃。胸片显示肺叶实变。因病情恶化而行气管插管，放置中心静脉置管，开始液体复苏。据患者丈夫陈述，一个星期前他们刚从泰国休假回来。

2. 临床问题

近期旅行会改变你的经验抗菌素的选择吗？

3. 答案

患者要同时使用针对类鼻疽和类鼻疽伯克氏菌类鼻疽的抗生素。

4. 感染途径包括直接接触、吸入或食入细菌。

5. 类鼻疽伯克氏菌在泰国和澳大利亚北部极为流行，而类鼻疽在美洲、亚洲和澳大利亚的其他区域也有发生。

6. 最常见的临床表现为肺部感染、脓肿形成和菌血症。

7. 没有经验的实验室在培养该细菌时会很困难，它经常被误诊。

8. 治疗：主要是 10～14 天疗程的头孢他啶或碳青霉烯类抗生素。

9. 患者恢复后，为彻底清除细菌，还需要服用 3～6 个月的复方新诺明。

10. 要点

对有严重感染和近期到流行区旅游的患者，确诊前应给予头孢他啶或碳青霉烯类抗生素。

参考文献：

Wiersinga WJ, Currie BJ, Peacock SJ. Melioidosis. N Engl J Med. 2012；367（11）：1035 -1044.

作者：**Jenny Reifel Saltzberg**

感染性疾病

115. Salmonellosis-What you need to know

1. General Information:

1) Salmonella: gram-negative rod-shaped bacilli.

2) S/S: diarrhea (often bloody), fever and abdominal cramping.

3) Incubation: 12 – 24hrs.

4) duration: 4 – 7 d.

5) Generally resolves without treatment. Antibiotics prolong bacterial shedding and thus only recommended in severely ill patients (high fever, severe diarrhea/dehydration, sepsis), the very young, and the very old.

2. Area of the world affected:

Worldwide, especially in developing countries.

3. Relevance to the US physician

As of Oct. 7th, 278 people infected in the most recent US outbreak, thought to be related to chicken from Foster Farms. Many of these strains of Samonella were drug-resistant.

4. Bottom Line:

Suspect Salmonellosis in patients with appropriate exposure and symptoms, give supportive care for most, only give antibiotics to severely ill patients after sending blood and stool culture and sensitivities.

Author: Andrea Tenner

115.沙门氏菌病，你需要知道什么？

1.一般资料

1）沙门菌：革兰氏阴性杆菌。

2）症状/体征：腹泻（常为血性）、发热和腹部绞痛。

3）潜伏期：12~24 小时。

4）病程：4~7 天。

5）一般无需治疗即可痊愈。抗生素可延长细菌排出，因此只建议在重症患者（高烧，严重腹泻/脱水，败血症）、很年轻和很老的患者中应用。

2.影响的区域

世界范围内，特别是在发展中国家。

3.与美国医生相关：

截至 2013 年 10 月 7 日，在美国已有 278 人感染，一般认为与 Foster 农场鸡有关。这些沙门氏菌的许多菌株都是耐药的。

4.要点

对有接触史和症状的可疑沙门氏菌病患者，主要是支持治疗，只有对那些做过血液和粪便培养及敏感试验的重症患者才给予抗生素治疗。

参考文献：

http：//www.cdc.gov/salmonella/heidelberg－10－13/index.html

作者：**Andrea Tenner**

感
染
性
疾
病

116. Listeria Infection

1. General Information:

1) Listeria can cause serious infections in vulnerable groups: adults > 65 years old, pregnant women, newborns, immunocompromised.

2) In a recent CDC report, infection with Listeria was associated with a 20% mortality rate.

2. Clinical Presentation:

1) History of cantaloupe, soft cheese, or raw produce ingestion.

2) Non-specific symptoms: fever, myalgias, occasionally preceded by GI symptoms.

3) Can have headache, stiff neck, confusion, AMS, miscarriage or stillbirth in pregnant women.

3. Diagnosis:

1) Blood, CSF, or amniotic fluid culture showing Listeria monocytogenes.

2) Listeria is a reportable disease.

4. Treatment:

1) Ampicillin and Penicillin G are the drugs of choice.

2) Add gentamycin in CSF infection, endocarditis, the immunocompromised, and neonates.

5. Bottom Line:

Listeria infections have a high mortality rate and can be found worldwide. Suspect in patients who have febrile syndromes and travel to areas where they may consume unpasteurized cheese.

Author: Andrea Tenner

116. 李斯特菌感染

1. 一般资料

1) 李斯特菌在65岁以上的老人、孕妇、新生儿和免疫功能低下等等易感人群中能引起严重感染。

2) 疾病控制中心(CDC)最近的报告显示：李斯特菌感染的死亡率可达20%。

2. 临床表现

1) 有食用香瓜、软奶酪或生农产品史。

2) 非特异性症状：发热，肌肉疼痛，之前有可能偶尔出现胃肠道症状。

3) 可出现头痛、颈项强直、神志不清、意识改变、孕妇流产或死胎。

3. 诊断

1) 血液、脑脊液或羊水培养出单核细胞增生李斯特菌。

2) 李斯特菌是一种要上报的疾病。

4. 治疗方法

1) 氨苄青霉素和青霉素 G 为首选药物；

2) 对于颅内感染、心内膜炎免疫功能低下者和新生儿应添加庆大霉素。

5. 要点

李斯特菌感染死亡率高，可在世界各地出现。对可能食用未经高温消毒奶酪并有发热症状的旅游者，要怀疑此疾病。

参考文献：

Older Americans, pregnant women face highest risk from Listeria food poisoning. http://www.cdc.gov/media/releases/2013/p0604-listeria-poisoning.html

作者：Andrea Tenner

感染性疾病

117. Tdap Recommended for all Patients 65 Years and Older

1. The two available Tetanus/reduced diphtheria toxoid/acellular pertussis (Tdap) vaccine products in the U. S. are Boostrix and Adacel. Neither were originally approved in older adults age 65 and older. Boostrix received FDA-approval for use in this age group in July 2011, but Adacel never has.

2. However, in June 2012 ACIP issued new guidance recommending Tdap for all adults age 65 years and older.

3. "When feasible, Boostrix should be used for adults aged 65 years and older; however, ACIP concluded that either vaccine administered to a person 65 years or older is immunogenic and would provide protection. A dose of either vaccine may be considered valid."

4. Bottom line: Regardless of which Tdap product is stocked at your institution, both are considered safe to use in adults 65 years and older.

Author: Bryan Hayes

117. 破伤风－白喉－百日咳疫苗 可用于 65 岁以上的患者

1. 在美国，破伤风－白喉－百日咳疫苗（Tdap）有两种剂型，Boostrix（白喉、破伤风和高纯度无细胞百日咳抗原的加强型疫苗）和 Adacel（抗白喉、百日咳、脊髓灰质炎和破伤风感染的加强型疫苗），二者起初均不能用于 65 岁以上患者。2011 年 7 月，美国食品药品监督管理局（FDA）批准了 Boostrix 在这一年龄段患者中的应用，而 Adacel 未获批准。

2. 但在 2012 年 6 月，美国免疫疫苗实践顾问委员会（ACIP）发表了一个新的指南，建议两种 Tdap 疫苗都可用于 65 岁以上患者。

3. "如有可能，对 65 岁以上患者要使用 Boostrix。但是，ACIP 认为在 65 岁以上患者中应用任何一种疫苗都会产生免疫效应并起到保护作用。一个剂量的任何一种疫苗都可以认为是有效的。"

4. 要点

根据医疗机构药房 Tdap 疫苗储备情况，两种疫苗都可以安全的用于 65 岁以上患者。

参考文献：

Centers for Disease Control and Prevention（CDC），"Updated Recommendations for Use of Tetanus Toxoid，Reduced Diphtheria Toxoid，and Acellular Pertussis（Tdap）Vaccine in Adults Aged 65 Years and Older - Advisory Committee on Immunization Practices（ACIP），" MMWR Morb Mortal Wkly Rep，2012，61(25)：468－70.[PMID 22739778]

作者：Bryan Hayes

感染性疾病

118. Updated Guidelines for Acute Uncomplicated Cystitis in Women

1. In 2011, updated treatment guidelines were published for acute uncomplicated cystitis and pyelonephritis in women. The recommendations differ from the previous iteration due to increased E. Coli resistance.

2. Cystitis (recommendations in order of preference)

1) Nitrofurantoin 100 mg BID X 5 days.

2) Bactrim DS 1 tab BID X 3 days (not recommended when resistance rate is >20%).

3) Fosfomycin.

4) Fluoroquinolones not recommended as first-line therapy due to " propensity for collateral damage".

5) Beta-lactam agents, including amoxicillin-clavulanate, cefdinir, cefaclor, and cefpodoxime-proxetil, in 3 – 7 – day regimens are appropriate choices for therapy when other recommended agents cannot be used. Other beta-lactams, such as cephalexin, are less well studied but may also be appropriate in certain settings.

3. Take home points:

1) Be familiar with your institution's antibiogram.

2) Use nitrofurantoin first-line for uncomplicated cystitis in women (it is contraindicated with CrCl <60 mL/min).

3) Consider beta-lactams such as Augmentin or Vantin (cefpodoxime) in patient's with kidney injury.

Author: Bryan Hayes

美
国
急
诊
临
床
必
知
200
招

118. 女性急性无合并症膀胱炎治疗的新指南

1.2011 年发表了女性急性无合并症膀胱炎治疗的新指南,由于大肠杆菌耐药性的增加,新的指南和过去的有所不同。

2.膀胱炎(按推荐顺序)

1)呋喃妥因 100 mg,一天两次,共五天。

2)复方新诺明,1 片,一天两次,共三天(如耐药率超过 20% 则不推荐)。

3)磷霉素。

4)氟喹诺酮类由于其副作用而不作为一线药推荐。

5)包括阿莫西林 - 克拉维酸钾、头孢地尼、头孢克洛、头孢泊肟酯在内的 3~7天 β 内酰胺类抗生素方案在无其他药物可用的情况下也可考虑。对其他的 β 内酰胺类抗生素如头孢胺苄的研究不多,在某种情况下也可应用。

3.要点

1)要熟悉本院的抗菌谱;

2)对女性没有合并症的膀胱炎首选呋喃妥因(肌酐清除率 <60 mL/min 时禁用);

3)如患者有肾损伤,可用阿莫西林克拉维酸钾或头孢泊肟。

参考文献:

Gupta K, et al. International Clinical Practice Guidelines for the Treatment of Acute Uncomplicated Cystitis and Pyelonephritis in Women: A 2010 Update by the Infectious Diseases Society of America and the European Society for Microbiology and Infectious Diseases. Clinical Infectious Diseases 2011; 52(5): e103 – e120.

作者: Bryan Hayes

感染性疾病

119. PD-associated peritonitis

1. Peritoneal dialysis (PD) is a commonly used form of dialysis for pediatric patients with end-stage renal disease, particularly in children less than five years of age.

2. One well known complication to this mode of dialysis is PD-associated peritonitis.

3. Children may present with fever, abdominal pain and a cloudy dialysate.

4. If peritonitis is suspected, obtain sample of dialysate fluid and send for cell count, Gram's stain and culture.

5. Cell count in PD-associated peritonitis is usually WBC >100 with >50% neutrophils.

6. Both gram-positive and gram-negative organisms are involved with PD-associated peritonitis. Keep both MRSA and Pseudomonas in mind.

7. In the ED, empiric therapy should cover both gram-positive and gram-negative organisms. Initiate antibiotic therapy with vancomycin and either a third-generation cephalosporin (ceftazidime) or aminoglycoside, respectively.

8. For PD-associated peritonitis, intraperitoneal (IP) administration of antibiotics is preferred over IV.

Author: Vikramjit Gill

119.腹膜透析相关地腹膜炎

1.腹膜透析是治疗儿童晚期肾病中的常用透析方法,尤其对于 5 岁以下的小儿。

2.这种透析最常见合并症是腹透相关性腹膜炎。

3.患儿表现为发热、腹部疼痛和透析液浑浊。

4.如怀疑为腹膜炎,应留取透析液查细胞计数、革兰染色和培养。

5.在腹透相关性腹膜炎中,白细胞超过 $100 \times 10^9/L$,中性粒细胞比例超过 50%。

6.腹膜透析相关性腹膜炎可由革兰氏阳性或阴性致病菌引起,要警惕 MRSA 和绿脓杆菌感染。

7.在急诊科,经验性治疗要覆盖革兰氏阳性和阴性菌。初始治疗可用万古霉素联合三代头孢(头孢他啶)或氨基糖苷类。

8.对于腹透相关地腹膜炎,抗生素腹腔内注射要优于静脉注射。

参考文献:

Li PK, et al. Peritoneal Dialysis-Related Infections Recommendations: 2010 Update. Peritoneal Dialysis International, Vol. 30, pp. 393 – 423.

Fadrowski JJ, et al. Children on long-term dialysis in the United States: findings from the 2005 ESRD clinical performance measures project. Am J Kidney Dis. 2007; 50(6): 958.

作者: **Vikramjit Gill**

感染性疾病

120. Neisseria meningitides?

1. This winter season has brought a rise in influenza and RSV activity in Maryland and in many parts of the country. It is also important to remember other potentially lethal infections that are prevalent in the winter and early spring months, such as Neisseria meningitidis. In fact, a recent study2 showed a potential increase in meningococcal disease when influenza and RSV activity is high.

2. What: Encapsulated, gram-negative diplococcus.

3. Where: Found in nasopharyngeal secretions, carrier rates 2 – 30% in normal populations.

4. Who: Age of incidence has 2 peaks: children < 2 years old, teens 15 – 19 years old Young adults who live in shared housing, such as college dorms and military recruits.

5. Clinical Presentation: Early non-specific symptoms of URI, fever, malaise, myalgias Meningitis: non-specific prodrome + headache, stiff neck (not found in younger children who often present atypically with irritability and/or vomiting) Meningococcemia: above symptoms + hypotension + petechial rash (>60% of patients).

6. Treatment: Early (!) antibiotics: 3rd generation cephalosporins (<3mo: cefotaxime; older infants, children, and teens: ceftriaxone); PCN G is antibiotic of choice for susceptible isolates Early and aggressive management of shock.

7. Prevention: Tetravalent vaccine, MCV4 (Menactra, Menveo), available for serogroups A, C, Y and W – 135 is given routinely at age 11 – 12 years old with an additional booster at 16 – 17 years old. MCV4 does not protect against serogroup B which accounts for 30% of infections.

Author: Lauren Rice

美
国
急
诊
临
床
必
知
200
招

120. 脑膜炎奈瑟菌

1. 这个冬季，马里兰和美国的许多地区出现了较高的流感和呼吸道合胞病毒的感染。同时我们也要记住其他在冬天和早春流行的潜在的致命感染，如脑膜炎奈瑟菌。事实上，最近研究显示：当流感和呼吸道合胞病毒活跃时，流脑发病呈升高趋势。

2. 是什么：具有夹膜的革兰氏阴性双球菌。

3. 在哪里：存在于鼻咽分泌物中，在正常人群中的携带率为 2% ~ 30%。

4. 易感人群：感染年龄的两个高峰期：两岁以内的儿童；15 ~ 19 岁住在集体宿舍（大学宿舍或军营）的青少年。

5. 临床表现：早期为非特异的上呼吸道症状，如发热、乏力、肌肉酸痛。脑膜炎：不特异的前期表现和头痛，颈项强直（在小儿中不常见，他们多表现为不特异的易怒和/或呕吐）。脑膜炎球菌血症：60% 以上的患者有上述症状并伴有低血压和出血性皮疹。

6. 治疗：早期抗生素：三代头孢（小于 3 个月：头孢噻肟；大一点的婴儿、儿童和青少年：头孢曲松）；青霉素 G 对敏感的菌群是早期和抢救休克时的首选的抗生素。

7. 预防：四价流行性脑脊髓膜炎疫苗（血清 A，C，Y 和 W – 135 型） – MCV4 常规在 11 ~ 12 岁时接种，并在 16 ~ 17 岁时增强。MCV4 对占 30% 感染的 B 型无效。

参考文献：

Cross JT, Hannaman RA. Infectious Disease. MedStudy Pediatrics Board Review Core Curriculum：5th edition. 2012；5 – 11.

Jansen AG, Sanders EA, VAN DER Ende A, VAN Loon AM, Hoes AW, Hak E. Invasive pneumococcal and meningococcal disease：association with influenza virus and respiratory syncytial virus activity?. Epidemiol Infect. Nov 2008；136(11)：1448 – 54.

Javid MH. Meningococcemia. Available at http：//emedicine. medscape. com/article/221473. Medscape Reference. Last updated Aug. 2. 2012.

作者：**Lauren Rice**

感染性疾病

121. PPD positive?

Background Information:

1. Active tuberculosis (TB) develops in 5 – 10% of individuals who become infected with M. tuberculosis, typically after a latency period of 6 – 18 months (but sometimes decades later). Compliance with the 9 month self-supervised isoniazid (INH) regimen has been poor with completion rates < 60%. Until recently, daily rifampin for 4 – 6 months has been the only alternative when the bacterium is resistant or INH cannot be used.

2. Pertinent Study Design and Conclusions:

1) Another rifamycin class antibiotic, Rifapentine (RPT) is approved for MDR-TB but had not been approved for latent TB treatment.

2) Recent RCTs show 12 weekly doses of INH-RPT administered as directly observed therapy (DOT) are efficacious in preventing active disease and are better tolerated.

3. CDC now recommends the 12 week INH-RPT DOT regimen as an equal alternative to 9 months of self supervised daily INH in patients aged > 12 years who have a high likelihood of developing active TB.

4. Bottom LIne:

A substantially shorter course of therapy with INH-RPT is now the recommended treatment for latent TB.

Author: Emilie J. B. Calvello

121. 结核菌素试验阳性?

1. 背景资料

结核分枝杆菌感染的患者中有 5% ~ 10% 会发展成活动性结核,通常在感染后 6 ~ 18 个月(但有时会在几十年后)。自我监督下的 9 个月 INH 方案的完成率不高,在 60% 以下。对于细菌耐药和不适用 INH 的患者,服用 4 ~ 6 个月利福平的方案是唯一的选择。

2. 相关的实验设计和结论

1)另外一个利福霉素类的抗生素利福喷丁(RPT)已被批准用于多药物耐药性的结核治疗,但还不能用于潜伏期结核的治疗。

2)最近临床试验结果显示,为期 12 周的 INH-RPT 在直接监督下服用可非常有效地防止活动性结核,并具有更好的耐受性。

3. 美国疾病控制中心建议对有可能发展成活动性结核的 12 岁以上的患者采用直接 12 周 INH-RPT 直接监督疗法来替代自行监督 9 个月的 INH 方案。

4. 要点

可以用相对短疗程的 INH-RPT 方案来治疗潜伏期的结核。

参考文献:

CDC. Recommendations for use of an isoniazid-rifapentine regimen with direct observation to treat latent Mycobacterium tuberculosis infection. MMWR Morb Mortal Wkly Rep, 2011 Dec 9; 60(48): 1650 – 1653.

作者: **Emilie J. B. Calvello**

感
染
性
疾
病

122. HIV viral suppression initiated in ED

1. Background Information:

Combination antiretroviral therapy (cART) reduces HIV-associated morbidities and mortalities but cannot cure infection. Recent literature has suggested that early initiation of cART with primary infection can lead to "functional cure" for HIV infected patients with suppressed viremia and delayed progression to clinical symptoms.

2. Pertinent Study Design and Conclusion:

(1) Researchers studied 14 patients whose treatment with combination antiretrovirals began soon after exposure to HIV. The patients' viral loads became undetectable within roughly 3 months, and treatment was interrupted after about 3 years.

(2) The patients were found to have very low viral loads and stable CD4 – cell counts after several years without therapy. The researchers estimate that about 15% of those treated early could achieve similar results.

3. Bottom Line:

Have a high suspicion of acute HIV syndrome in the ED (fever, rash, pharyngitis, lymphadenopathy) and test properly (viral load NOT ELISA) to identify patients who may benefit from early, rapid initiation of cART.

Author: Emilie J. B. Calvello

122. 在急诊科开始 HIV 病毒抑制治疗

1. 背景资料

抗逆转录病毒联合疗法(cART)可以减少 HIV 相关的并发症的发病率和死亡率,但不能治愈 HIV 感染。最新文献提示对原发性感染的患者早期使用 cART 可以"功能性治愈"感染 HIV 的患者,控制病毒血症和延缓临床症状的发展。

2. 有关研究设计和结论

1)研究人员研究了 14 例在感染艾滋病毒后很快接受抗逆转录病毒药物联合治疗患者,患者的病毒载量在大约 3 个月内就检测不到了,3 年后停止治疗。

2)停药几年后,患者具有非常低的病毒载量和稳定的 CD4 细胞计数。研究人员估计,约 15% 的早期治疗患者可以达到类似的效果。

3. 要点

在急诊科,对高度怀疑具有急性艾滋病毒感染综合征表现(发热、皮疹、淋巴结肿大、咽炎)的患者需适当检查(病毒载量而不是 ELISA),以识别那些可能会受益于早期和快速 cART 治疗的患者。

参考文献:

Sáez-Cirión A, Bacchus C, Hocqueloux L, Avettand-Fenoel V, Girault I, et al. (2013) Post-Treatment HIV-1 Controllers with a Long-Term Virological Remission after the Interruption of Early Initiated Antiretroviral Therapy ANRS VISCONTI Study. PLoS Pathog 9(3): e1003211.

作者: **Emilie J. B. Calvello**

感
染
性
疾
病

外科与外伤
Surgery and Trauma

123. Traumatic Hemorrhage Shock

1. When managing the critically ill patient with traumatic hemorrhagic shock, the primary objectives are to stop bleeding, maintain tissue perfusion and oxygen delivery, and limit organ dysfunction.

2. Pearls to consider when resuscitating these patients include:

1) In the patient without brain injury, target an SBP of 80 – 100 mm Hg until major bleeding has been controlled.

2) Limit aggressive fluid resuscitation.

3) Avoid delays in blood and blood component transfusion. Transfuse early. Though the optimal ratio remains controversial, most transfuse PRBCs and FFP in a 1 : 1 ratio.

4) Consider point-of-care testing, such as thromboelastography (TEG), to assess the degree of coagulopathy and guide transfusion strategies.

5) Consider the use of tranexamic acid.

Author: Michael Winters

123. 创伤性出血性休克

1. 在处理创伤性出血性休克危重患者时，主要的目的是止血、维持组织灌注和供氧及减少器官损伤。

2. 对于这样的患者复苏的精髓包括：

1) 对没有脑损伤的患者，在大出血没有控制前，维持收缩压在 80～100 mmHg。

2) 限制性液体复苏。

3) 不要延误输血或血液成分，尽快输血！虽然还没有明确的比例，全血和血浆的比例应该为 1:1。

4) 考虑床旁检测，如凝血弹性描记法确定凝血障碍的程度并指导输血计划。

5) 考虑用氨甲环酸。

参考文献：

Bougle A, et al. Resuscitative strategies in traumatic hemorrhagic shock. Annals of Intensive Care 2013; 3.

作者：**Michael Winters**

外科与外伤

124. Trauma Fluid Resuscitation?

1. Pre-hospital

1) One study found urban trauma patients only receive 17 min and 380mL of IVF before arriving at the hospital.

2) One study of patients with penetrating trauma found no statistical difference in mortality between those who received < 100mL IVF vs > 100mL IVF.

3) Large recent study of 776, 000 patients showed a death OR of 1. 1 in patients who received IVF pre-hospital.

4) More important is to get patients to the hospital quickly than to take the time to place IV in field.

2. ED management

1) Permissive hypotension leads to better outcomes!

2) Giving lots of IVF leads to increased BP and increased blood loss, which includes loss of clotting factors. This contributes to the trauma "triad of death: " coagulopathy, hypothermia, and acidosis.

3) In patients with significant blood loss and persistent hypotension/AMS despite 1L IVF, move quickly to massive transfusion protocol (1 : 1 : 1 PRBC, FFP, platelets), leads to better outcomes.

4) ABC score (1 point for each, higher the points the higher the likelihood of benefit from massive transfusion protocol): Penetrating injury, Tachycardia (HR > 120), Hypotension (SBP < 90), Positive FAST.

5) CAVEAT: No permissive hypotension in patients with TBI!!!

3. CCM in ED

1) Lactate -if going the wrong direction, give more blood, not pressors or crystalloid.

2) Check ionized calcium when giving bloods.

3) Keep patient warm, Continuous rectal temp monitor, In-line IV warmers, Humidified air for vent.

4) Sedate and control pain (think fentanyl).

5) Complications: Early ARDS or transfusion related acute lung injury and ACS.

Authors: J. V. Nable, Michael Bond, & John Greenwood

外
科
与
外
伤

124. 创伤的液体复苏

1. 院前

1）研究指出，城市外伤患者平均需要 17 分钟送到医院并在到达医院前仅仅接受 380 mL 的静脉给液。

2）另一研究指出，穿透伤患者在接受静脉给液 100 mL 以下和以上的患者间的死亡率没有统计学差异。

3）最新的一个包括了 776000 例患者的报告指出，院前接受静脉输液的患者的死亡比值比是 1.1。

4）比在现场花时间进行静脉给液更重要的是尽快将患者转运到医院。

2. 急诊科治疗

1）允许性低血压预后较好！

2）静脉输液过多可在升高血压的同时增加失血量，包括凝血因子的丢失。进而导致外伤"死亡三要素"的产生：凝血功能紊乱、低温和酸中毒。

3）对于大失血和输 1 升液体后血压仍低或神志不清的患者，积极采用快速大量输血方案（全血、血浆和血小板按 1∶1∶1 的比例输注），预后较好。

4）预测输血评分标准（每项一分，分越高提示大量输血方案改善预后的可能性越大）：穿透伤，心动过速（心率超过 120 次/分），低血压（收缩压低于 90 mm-Hg），FAST 腹部超声阳性。

5）注意：允许性低血压在脑外伤中不适用！！！

3. 危重病医学在急诊科的应用

1）监测乳酸：如升高，多输血，不要用升压药或晶体液。

2）输血时要监测游离钙。

3）保持患者体温：持续监测直肠温度，静脉输液温化器，呼吸机气体雾化。

4）镇静和疼痛控制（可考虑用芬太尼）。

5）注意合并症：早期的呼吸困难窘迫综合征或与输血有关的肺损伤和急性冠脉综合征。

参考文献：

Dalton AM. Prehospital intravenous fluid replacement in trauma: an outmoded concept? Journal of the Royal Society of Medicine 1995; 88(4): 213 – 16.

Yaghoubian A, Lewis RJ, Putnam B, De Virgilio C. Reanalysis of prehospital intravenous fluid administration in patients with penetrating truncal injury and field hypotension. American Surgeon 2007; 73(10) – 1027 – 30.

Haut ER, Kalish BT, Cotton BA et al. Prehospital intravenous fluid administration is associated with higher mortality in trauma patients: a National Trauma Data Bank analysis. Annals of Surgery 2011; 253(2): 371 – 7.

Bickell WH, Wall MJ Jr., Pepe PE et al. Immediate versus delayed fluid resuscitation for hypotensive patients with penetrating torso injuries. New England Journal of Medicine 1994; 331(17): 1105 – 9.

作者: **J. V. Nable, Michael Bond, & John Greenwood**

外
科
与
外
伤

125. Massive Transfusion Pearls

1. Massive transfusion (MT) is defined as the transfusion of at least 10 U of packed red blood cells (PRBCs) within 24 hours.

2. While the optimal ratio of PRBCs, FFP, and platelets is not known, most use a 1 : 1 : 1 ratio.

3. Though scoring systems have been published to identify patients who may benefit from MT (ABC, TASH, McLaughlin), they have not been shown to be superior to clinical judgment.

4. A few pearls when implementing massive transfusion for the patient with traumatic shock:

1) Monitor temperature and aggressively treat hypothermia.

2) Monitor fibrinogen levels and replace with cryoprecipitate if needed.

3) Monitor calcium and potassium. MT can induce hypocalcemia and hyperkalemia.

Author: Michael Winters

125. 大量输血注意事项

1. 大量输血(MT)的定义是在 24 小时内至少输 10 个单位的浓缩红细胞(PRBCs)。

2. 输 PRBCs、冻干血浆(FFP)和血小板的最佳比例还不清楚,最常使用的比例为 1:1:1。

3. 虽然已有可识别对 MT 受益患者的评分系统(ABC,TASH,McLaughlin),但他们都并不比临床判断好。

4. 在给创伤性休克患者实施大量输血时,有几个注意事项:

1)监测体温并积极治疗体温过低。

2)监测纤维蛋白原水平,必要时输冷沉淀。

3)监测血钙和血钾。MT 可诱发低钙血症和高钾血症。

参考文献:

Elmer J, et al. Massive transfusion in traumatic shock. J Emerg Med 2013;44:829 – 838.

作者:**Michael Winters**

外科与外伤

126. Global Burden of Injuries

1. General Information:

1) Injuries are responsible for 10% of all deaths worldwide.

2) About 5.8 million people die from injuries worldwide every year.

3) Injuries kill 32% more people around the world than malaria, tuberculosis, and HIV/AIDS combined.

4) Injuries have an immeasurable impact on the families and communities affected.

5) They are responsible for about 16% of all disabilities.

6) Road traffic injuries are the leading cause of injury related deaths among young people, aged 15 – 29 years. Available global cost estimates show that the cost of road injuries annually is about US $ 518 billion.

7) More than 90% of deaths that result from road traffic injuries occur in low- and middle-income countries.

8) Road traffic crashes cost most countries 1 – 2% of their Gross National Product (GNP).

2. Relevance to the EM Physician:

Although road traffic injury deaths have decreased in some high-income countries, by 2030 it is predicted that they will be the fifth leading cause of death worldwide, and the seventh leading cause of Disability Adjusted Life Years (DALY) lost.

3. Bottom Line:

Developing trauma and acute care capacities in low and middle-income countries is of utmost importance to mitigate the global burden of injuries.

Author: Andrea Tenner

126. 外伤的全球危害

1. 一般资料

1）外伤占全球所有死亡的 10%。

2）每年全世界约 580 万人死于外伤。

3）世界各地因外伤死亡的人数要比因疟疾、肺结核、艾滋病死亡的总和多 32% 以上。

4）外伤对家庭和社区有不可估量的影响。

5）由此致残的人数占所有残障人数的 16% 左右。

6）道路交通事故是 15~29 岁年轻人外伤致死的首要原因。现有的全球成本预测表明，每年交通事故外伤的成本大约是 5180 亿美元。

7）因交通事故导致的死亡 90% 以上发生在低收入和中等收入国家。

8）大多数国家的交通事故成本超过其国民生产总值（GNP）的 1%~2%。

2. 与急诊医师有关

虽然一些高收入国家的道路交通事故死亡人数有所下降，但到 2030 年，它将成为全世界第五大死因和伤残调整寿命年（DALY）缩短的第七大原因。

3. 要点

提升低收入和中等收入国家创伤和急症抢救能力对于缓解全球外伤负担是极其重要的。

参考文献：

World Health Organization，Global status report on road safety，2013

http：//www. who. int/violence_injury_prevention/road_safety_status/2013/en/

World Health Organization，Injuries Violence：The Facts，2010

http：//www. who. int/violence_injury_prevention/key_facts/en/

作者：Andrea Tenner

外科与外伤

293

127. Do Monitors in severe traumatic brain injury Matter?

1. Management of patients with severe traumatic brain injury (TBI) typically involves the use of invasive intra-parenchymal pressure monitors. Although use of these monitors is recommended by TBI management guidelines, good quality evidence of benefit is lacking.

2. A recently published study evaluated the outcomes of TBI patients using a management protocol incorporating either an intracranial pressure (ICP) monitor compared to use of the clinical exam PLUS serial neuroimaging; a total of 324 patients were prospectively randomized into either group.

3. The primary study outcome was a composite of survival, impaired consciousness, and functional status at both three and six months.

4. The results of the study did not show a significant difference in the:

1) Primary outcome.

2) Median length of ICU stay.

3) Distribution of serious adverse events.

5. Bottom line: This study suggests that clinical exam PLUS serial neuroimaging may perform as well as invasive intra-parenchymal monitors for guiding therapy in TBI patients.

Author: Haney Mallemat

127. 严重的创伤性脑损伤需要监测颅压吗？

1. 严重的创伤性脑损伤(TBI)通常要使用侵入性颅内压力监测，虽然 TBI 处理指南中建议进行监测，但该监测缺乏足够有力的支持证据。

2. 一篇最新发表的文章对 TBI 患者在用颅内压监测和用临床检查包括系列脑影像方案的预后进行了评价，将 324 名患者进行前瞻性地随机分组。

3. 主要的研究指标包括患者在 3 和 6 个月时的生存率、神志障碍和功能状态。

4. 研究结果显示，在如下几个方面没有明显差别：

1）主要预后指标；

2）平均 ICU 住院时间；

3）严重的恶性事件的发生。

5. 要点

这个研究显示，在 TBI 患者的治疗中，临床检查加上系列神经影像与侵入性颅内压监测有同样的作用。

参考文献：

Chestnut，R. et al. A Trial of Intracranial-Pressure Monitoring in Traumatic Brain Injury. NEJM 2012 Dec 12.

作者：Haney Mallemat

外科与外伤

128. Frostbite Treatment

"Frozen in January, Amputate in June" – By Kinjal Sethuraman and Doug Sward

1. Frostbite can lead to major tissue damage even if initial presentation does not look so severe. Treatment is NOT the same as for burns.

2. Treatment of Major Frostbite:

1) Rapid rewarming ASAP of affected area in 40 Celsius degree water until area is thawed (pink and pliable). Logistics are difficult because you have to maintain a constant water temperature-but only if you can maintain same degree of warmth. Rewarming and refreezing will lead to inevitable tissue death.

2) Wound care, Aloe Vera, ASA.

3) DELAY surgery except in cases of sepsis or compartment syndrome.

3. CUTTING EDGE:

1) If less than 24 hours since injury, consider diagnostic angiography and intra-arterial TPA, and heparin infusion, Prostacyclin infusion.

2) Angiography and Bone Scan can be used to prognosticate clinical course.

3) Consider Hyperbaric Oxygen Therapy for moderate to severe frostbite- multiple case reports of significant improvement with HBOT even if delayed by several days.

4. Treatment of Minor Frostbite:

1) Rewarm area.

2) Ibuprofen.

3) Aloe Vera and dressing changes.

Author: Michael Bond

128.冻伤的治疗

"一月份冻伤,六月份截肢" – Kinjal Sethuraman 和 Doug Sward 医生。

1.冻伤可能导致严重的组织损伤,即使初期表现看起来不那么严重。治疗方法与烧伤不一样。

2.严重冻伤的治疗方法:

1)尽快将患处浸入 40℃ 的温水中快速复温,直到部位解冻(变得粉红和柔软)。一定要保持水温恒定,复温后再冻将导致不可避免的组织死亡。

2)伤口护理,芦荟,阿司匹林。

3)可以延迟手术,除非有败血症或骨筋膜室综合征。

3.新进展

1)如果冻伤后不到 24 小时,可考虑血管造影诊断及动脉给予抗栓塞药物,滴注肝素,静脉滴注前列环素。

2)血管造影和骨扫描可以用来判断临床进程。

3)对中度到严重的冻伤,可考虑高压氧治疗——有多个病例报告,即使延迟几天,高压氧治疗效果还是显著的。

4.轻微冻伤的治疗:

1)局部复温;

2)布洛芬;

3)芦荟和换药。

参考文献:

Frostbitehttp://www.ncbi.nlm.nih.gov/pubmed/21664561

作者:**Michael Bond**

外科与外伤

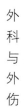

129. Isolated skull fractures in pediatrics

1. Pediatric patients with an isolated skull fracture and normal neurological exam have a low risk of neurosurgical intervention and outpatient follow up may be appropriate (assuming no suspicion of abuse and a reliable family).

2. In a study published in 2011, a retrospective review over a 5 year period at a level 1 trauma center showed that 1 out of 171 admitted patients with isolated skull fractures developed vomiting. This patient had a follow up CT showing a small extra-axial hematoma that did not require intervention. 58 patients were discharged from the ED within 4 hours.

3. You can also check out another recent article published in on the same topic this month!

Author: **Jennifer Guyther**

129. 儿科患者的单纯颅骨骨折

1. 一名神经系统检查正常的单纯颅骨骨折的小儿患者需要神经外科进行治疗的风险很低，门诊随访是可行的(假设没有虐待可能并且的家庭可信赖)。

2. 在 2011 年发表的一项研究中，通过 5 年的回顾性分析显示，在 1 级创伤中心的 171 例单纯颅骨骨折入院的患者中只有 1 人出现呕吐。随后的 CT 检查显示，该患者有一个小的轴外血肿，并不需要手术。58 例患者在 4 小时内从急诊科出院。

3. 您还可以查看同月在 Annals of Emergency Medicine 发表的另一篇文章！

参考文献：

Rollins et al. Neurologically intact children with an isolated skull fracture may be safely discharged after brief observation. Journal of Pediatric Surgery. Volume 26. Issue 7. 2011.

Mannix et al. Skull Fractures：Trends in Management in US Pediatric Emergency Departments. Annals of Emergency Medicine. Volume 64. Issue 4. 2013.

作者：Jennifer Guyther

外科与外伤

130. Pediatric Appendicitis Score

1. Risk stratisfication score introduced by Maden Samuel in 2002.

2. The Pediatric Appendicitis Score had a sensitivity of 1, specificity of 0.92, positive predictive value of 0.96, and negative predictive value of 0.99.

1) Signs:

(1) Right lower quadrant tenderness = 2 points

(2) Cough/Percussion/Hop RLQ tenderness = 1 point

(3) Pyrexia = 1 point

2) Symptoms:

(1) RLQ migration of pain = 1 point

(2) Anorexia = 1 point

(3) Nausea/Vomiting = 1 point

3) Laboratory Values:

(1) Leukocytosis = 2 points

(2) Polymorphonuclear neutrophilia = 1 point

3. Scores of 4 or less are least likely to have acute appendicitis, while scores of 8 or more are most likely.

Author: Rose Chasm

130. 儿童阑尾炎评分标准

1. 在 2002 年 Maden Samuel 医生提出了阑尾炎危险因素评估标准。

2. 这个小儿阑尾炎评分标准的灵敏度为 1，特异性为 0.92，阳性预测值为 0.96，阴性预测值为 0.99。

1) 体征

(1) 右下腹压痛 = 2 分；

(2) 咳嗽/敲击/跳蹦加重右下腹疼痛 = 1 分；

(3) 发热 = 1 分。

2) 症状

(1) 转移性右下腹痛 = 1 分；

(2) 厌食 = 1 分；

(3) 恶心/呕吐 = 1 分。

3) 实验室检查

(1) 白细胞增多 = 2 分；

(2) 中性粒细胞 = 1 分。

3. 少于 4 分的患者患有急性阑尾炎的可能性很低，而 8 分以上的可能性是最高的。

参考文献：

Samuel M. Pediatric Appendicits Score[J]. J Pedia Surg, 2002, 37：877 - 881.

作者：Rose Chasm

外科与外伤

131. Concussion in sport

"When can my child get back out on the field doc?"

1. Return to play(RTP)

1)Concussion symptoms should be resolved before returning to exercise.

2)A RTP progression involves a gradual, step-wise increase in physical demands, sports-specific activities and the risk for contact.

3)If symptoms occur with activity, the progression should be halted and restarted at the preceding symptom-free step.

4)RTP after concussion should occur only with medical clearance from a licenced healthcare provider trained in the evaluation and management of concussions.

2. Short-term risks of premature RTP

The primary concern with early RTP is decreased reaction time leading to an increased risk of a repeat concussion or other injury and prolongation of symptoms.

3. Long-term effects

1)There is an increasing concern that head impact exposure and recurrent concussions contribute to long-term neurological sequelae.

2)Some studies have suggested an association between prior concussions and chronic cognitive dysfunction. Large-scale epidemiological studies are needed to more clearly define risk factors and causation of any long-term neurological impairment.

Author: Brian Corwell

131. 脑震荡与体育运动

"医生，我的孩子什么时候能回到运动场?"

1. 恢复运动

1) 脑震荡症状完全消失后才能恢复运动。

2) 恢复运动的进展过程要循序渐进地增加从生理需求、体育专项活动到有接触的风险的运动。

3) 如随着活动的增加出现症状，那么要暂停活动，从前面没有症状的那一步重新开始。

4) 在脑震荡发生后恢复运动，一定要经过有执照的医疗服务人员的体检，这些人员应在脑震荡评估和处理方面经过专业培训。

2. 过早恢复运动的短期危险

由于反应时间的减慢，过早恢复运动可增加再次出现脑震荡或受其他外伤及延长症状时间的风险。

3. 过早恢复运动的长期危险

1) 脑部的撞击和再次脑震荡会造成长期的神经后遗症，这是一个越来越大的顾虑。

2) 一些研究认为脑震荡和慢性认知紊乱有一定的联系，要明确造成长期神经损伤的危险因素和原因，还需要大规模的流行病学的研究。

参考文献：

American Medical Society for Sports Medicine position statement：concussion in sport, 2013

作者：Brian Corwell

外科与外伤

303

132. Sports-related Concussion

1. Estimated 3. 8 million sport-related concussions per year (likely significantly higher due to underreporting).

2. Most patients recover within a 7 – 10 day period.

3. Children and teenagers require more time than college and professional athletes.

4. This "accepted" time for recovery is not scientifically established and there is a large degree of variability based on multiple factors including age (as above), sex & history of prior concussions.

5. Approximately 10% of athletes have persistent signs and symptoms beyond 2 weeks. (which may represent a prolonged concussion or the development of post-concussion syndrome)

6. During this time the patient should have complete rest from all athletic activities, close follow-up with PCP and be educated re concussions.

7. If practical, "cognitive rest" should also be prescribed. This is one of the most frequently neglected aspects of post-concussion care.

Author: Brian Corwell

132. 与体育运动有关的脑震荡

1. 每年大约会有 380 万与运动有关的脑震荡(实发率可能因为少报会更高)。

2. 多数患者将在 7~10 天内恢复。

3. 与大学生和专业运动员相比,儿童和青少年需要较长的时间恢复。

4. 这个"公认"的恢复期是没有任何科学依据的,会受许多因素(包括年龄、性别和既往脑震荡史)的影响并有很大的个体差异。

5. 大约有 10% 的运动员在两星期后还会有持续的体征和症状(可能提示过长的脑震荡或脑震荡后综合征的产生)。

6. 在这段时间内,患者应该注意休息,不参与任何体育活动,多向家庭医生咨询并加强脑震荡方面的教育。

7. 如果可行,还要强调"认知休息",这是在脑震荡后最容易被忽视的方面之一。

作者:Brian Corwell

外科与外伤

305

133. Hormonal Dysfunction in Neurologic Injury

1. In the critically ill patient with neurologic injury (SAH, TBI), the initial treatment focus is to maintain adequate cerebral perfusion pressure, control intracranial pressure, and limit secondary injury.

2. Once stabilized, however, it is important to consider endocrine dysfunction in the brain injured patient.

3. Endocrine dysfunction is common in neurologic injury and may lead to increased morbidity and mortality. In fact, over half of SAH patients develop acute dysfunction of the HPA, resulting in low growth hormone, ACTH, and TSH.

4. In addition to hormonal dysfunction, sodium abnormalities (i. e. hyponatremia) are present in up to 80% of critically ill SAH patients.

5. Consider hormonal replacement therapy (or hypertonic saline in cases of severe hyponatremia) for patients with evidence of endocrine dysfunction. For some, this therapy can be life-saving.

Author: Michael Winters

133. 神经系统损伤的激素紊乱

1. 在危重的神经系统损伤(蛛网膜下隙出血、外伤性脑损伤)患者中,初期治疗的焦点是保持足够的脑灌注压、控制颅内压和减少继发性损伤。

2. 但是,一旦病情稳定,对于脑损伤的患者就要关注内分泌紊乱的情况。

3. 内分泌紊乱在脑损伤中是常见的,并可增加合并症发病率和死亡率。事实上,超过一半以上的蛛网膜下隙出血的患者可出现急性下丘脑–垂体–肾上腺皮质轴功能紊乱,导致生长激素、促肾上腺皮质激素和促甲状腺激素水平降低。

4. 除了内分泌紊乱外,80%以上的严重蛛网膜下腔出血的患者可出现钠离子异常(如低钠血症)。

5. 有明显内分泌紊乱的患者可考虑用激素替代疗法(或在严重低钠时应用高渗盐水),这种方法可以挽救某些患者的生命。

参考文献:

Vespa PM. Hormonal dysfunction in neurocritical patients. Curr Opin Crit Care 2013;19:107 –112.

作者:Michael Winters

外科与外伤

134. Knee Injuries are Radiographs Needed

1. Many people know that the folks in Ottawa have come up with a rule to determine whether radiographs are needed in patients complaining of knee pain.

2. The Ottawa Knee rules that that radiographs are only required for knee injuries with any of the following:

1) Age 55 years or older.

2) isolated tenderness of patella.

3) tenderness at head of fibula.

4) inability to flex to 90'.

5) inability to bear weight both immediately and in the emergency department (4 steps).

3. Well another group in Pittsburgh have their own set of rules that were recently shown to be more specific with equal sensitivity.

4. The Pittsburgh decision rules state that radiographs are only needed if

There is a history of fall or blunt trauma AND (Patient is < 12 or > 50 years old OR Patient is unable to walk for weight bearing steps in the ED.)

5. So consider using the Pittsburgh or Ottawa Knee rules the next time you have a patient with knee pain to determine if those radiographs are really needed.

Author: Michael Bond

134. 膝关节受伤是否需要拍摄 X 线片

1. 很多人都知道，在渥太华的同行们提出了一个对膝关节疼痛的患者是否需要拍 X 线片的建议。

2. 渥太华膝关节规则建议膝关节损伤患者如满足下列条件之一，则需要拍 X 线片：

1）年龄≥55 岁；

2）髌骨压痛；

3）腓骨头压痛；

4）无法弯曲 90 度；

5）受伤后及在急诊科无法负重（走不到 4 步）。

3. 另外，另一组在匹兹堡的同行最近也发表了他们的规则，并被证明更特异并具有相同的敏感性。

4. 匹兹堡决策规则指出，只有在下列情况下才需要行 X 线片检查：

有跌倒或钝挫伤史并且患者 <12 岁或 >50 岁或患者在急诊科无法负重行走。

5. 所以在下一次面对膝关节疼痛患者时，可考虑使用匹兹堡或渥太华膝关节规则，以确定是否真正需要拍 X 线片。

参考文献：

Cheung TC, Tank Y, Breederveld RS, Tuinebreijer WE, de Lange-de Klerk ESM, MD RJD. Diagnostic accuracy and reproducibility of the Ottawa Knee Rule vs the Pittsburgh Decision Rule. Am J Emerg Med. Elsevier Inc; 2013 Feb 1; 1–5.

作者：**Michael Bond**

外科与外伤

135. Necrotizing Fasciitis

1. Necrotizing fasciitis (NF) is a rapidly progressive bacterial infection of the fascia with secondary necrosis of the subcutaneous tissue. In severe cases, the underlying muscle (i. e. , myositis) may be affected.

2. Risk factors for NF include immunosuppression (e. g. , transplant patients), HIV/AIDS, diabetes, etc.

3. There are three categories of NF:

Type I (poly-microbial infections).

Type II (Group A streptococcus; sometimes referred to as the "flesh-eating bacteria).

Type III (Clostridial myonecrosis; known as gas gangrene).

4. In the early stage of disease, diagnosis may be difficult; the physical exam sometimes does not reflect the severity of disease. Labs may be non-specific, but CT or MRI is important to diagnose and define the extent of the disease when planning surgical debridement.

5. Treatment should be aggressive and started as soon as the disease is suspected; this includes:

1) Aggressive fluid and/or vasopressor therapy.

2) Broad spectrum antibiotics covering for gram-positive, gram-negative, and anaerobic bacteria; clindamycin should be added initially as it suppresses certain bacterial toxin formation.

3) Emergent surgical consult for debridement.

6. Once the patient is stable, other treatments may include intravenous immunoglobulin and hyperbaric oxygen therapy.

Author: Haney Mallemat

135. 坏死性筋膜炎

1.坏死性筋膜炎（NF）是一种进展快速的细菌性筋膜感染，伴有继发性皮下组织坏死。在严重的情况下，筋膜下肌肉可能受到影响（即肌炎）。

2.NF 的危险因素包括免疫抑制剂的应用（例如，器官移植患者）、艾滋病毒感染/艾滋病和糖尿病等。

3.NF 有三型：

Ⅰ型（多微生物感染）；

Ⅱ型（A 组链球菌，有时也被称为"食肉菌"）；

Ⅲ型（梭菌性肌坏死，被称为气性坏疽）。

4.在疾病的早期阶段，诊断可能比较困难，体检有时并不反映疾病的严重程度。实验室检查可能无特异性，但当诊断或判断疾病是否需要进行外科清创时，CT 或 MRI 是很重要的。

5.一旦怀疑此病就要开始积极治疗，包括：

1）积极液体治疗和/或升压药治疗。

2）应用对革兰阳性菌、革兰阴性菌和厌氧菌都敏感的广谱抗生素；同时要加用克林霉素，因为它可抑制某些细菌毒素的产生。

3）外科紧急会诊以准备清创手术

6.一旦患者病情稳定，应采取包括静脉注射免疫球蛋白和高压氧治疗等其他治疗措施。

作者：**Haney Mallemat**

外科与外伤

311

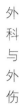

136. The End of Steroids for Acute Spinal Injury?

For those Emergency Physicians that work in hospitals where protocols still call for steroids for spinal cord injury, or work with neurosurgeons who still believe in the efficacy of such treatment, a recent statement in Neurosurgery would seem to put the issue to rest:

"Administration of methylprednisolone (MP) for the treatment of acute spinal cord injury (SCI) is not recommended. Clinicians considering MP therapy should bear in mind that the drug is not FDA approved for this application. There is no Class Ⅰ or Class Ⅱ medical evidence supporting the clinical benefit of MP in the treatment of acute SCI. Scattered reports of Class Ⅲ evidence claim inconsistent effects likely related to random chance or selection bias. However, Class Ⅰ, Ⅱ, and Ⅲ evidence exists that high-dose steroids are associated with harmful side effects including death."

Author: Feng Xiao

136. 是结束对急性脊髓损伤应用糖皮质激素的时候了

有些医院主张使用激素治疗神经损伤，对于工作在这些医院的急诊科医生和相信这种方法的神经外科医生来说，最近《神经外科》杂志的一个报告将结束对这一问题的疑惑：

"在治疗急性脊髓损伤（SCI）时，不推荐使用甲基强的松龙（MP），还在考虑用 MP 治疗的医师应该记住这种药物在 SCI 中的应用并没有得到 FDA 的批准。另外还没有 I 类或 II 类临床证据支持 MP 治疗急性脊髓损伤，仅有的几个 III 类证据报道的效果也不一致，可能与随机几率或选择性偏差有关。然而，确有 I 类、II类和 III 类的证据证实了高剂量的糖皮质激素的副作用，严重时甚至可致死亡。"

参考文献：

Hurlbert RJ, et al. Neurosurgery 2013 Mar; 72 Suppl 2：93 – 105

作者：**Feng Xiao**（肖锋）

外科与外伤

肾脏
Nephrology

137. Management of AKI

1. Managing Critically Ill Patients withAcute kidney injury (AKI).

2. AKI occurs in almost 50% of hospitalized patients and is an independent risk factor for mortality.

3. Updated guidelines have recently been published on the management of patients with AKI.

4. Pearls for the management of patients with, or at risk of, AKI include:

1) Optimize volume status and perfusion pressure.

2) Crystalloids preferred over colloids.

3) Consider vasopressors to maintain MAP >65 mm Hg.

4) Avoid nephrotoxic drugs.

5) Control co-factors.

6) Monitor intra-abdominal pressure.

7) Avoid hyperglycemia-target glucose <150 mg/dL.

Author: Michael Winters

137. 急性肾损伤的处理

1. 伴有急性肾损伤(AKI)的危重患者的治疗。

2. 50%的住院患者会出现 AKI，它是死亡率增加的独立危险因素。

3. 有关 AKI 患者的处理已有新的指南。

4. 处理 AKI 患者的要点有：

1) 改善容量状态和灌注压；

2) 晶体液优先于胶体液；

3) 可考虑血管升压药以维持平均动脉压大于 65 mmHg；

4) 避免肾毒性药物；

5) 控制并发因素；

6) 监测腹内压力；

7) 避免高血糖：目标血糖低于 8.3 mmol/L。

参考文献：

Brienza N，et al. Protocoled resuscitation and the prevention of acute kidney injury. Curr Opin Crit Care 2012；18：613 – 622.

Kidney Disease：Improving Global Outcomes（KDIGO）Acute Kidney Injury Work Group. KDIGO Clinical Practice Guideline for Acute Kidney Injury. Kidney Int 2012；2(S)：1 – 138.

作者：**Michael Winters**

肾
脏

138. NAC for Prevention of Contrast-Induced Nephropathy

1. A recent meta-analysis has called into question whether contrast-induced AKI even occurs after an IV dye load for radiologic imaging. [1] This conclusion is most certainly up for debate.

2. Irrespective of that conclusion, prevention of contrast-induced nephropathy is still important. Is there any benefit to using N-acetylcysteine over normal saline in the ED? Probably not according to a new study. [2]

1) The primary outcome was contrast-induced nephropathy, defined as an increase in creatinine level of 25% or 0.5 mg/dL, measured 48 to 72 hours after CT.

2) The authors found no reduction in contrast-induced nephropathy in patients who received NAC vs normal saline (about 7% in each group).

3) The important finding is that the contrast-induced nephropathy rate in patients receiving less than 1 L IV fluids in the ED was 13% compared to 3% for more than 1 L.

3. Conclusions

1) Contrast-induced AKI does happen after emergency CT.

2) NAC does not provide additional benefit over saline alone.

3) Giving more than 1 L of normal saline markedly reduces the risk.

Author: Bryan Hayes

138. N-乙酰半胱氨酸预防造影剂肾病

1.最近的一项 Meta 分析提出了一个问题，静脉注射用于放射影像学检查的造影剂可造成急性肾损伤，当然这个结论是有争议的。

2.无论这一结论如何，预防造影剂肾病的发生仍然是重要的。在急诊科应用 N-乙酰半胱氨酸(NAC)会比生理盐水有效吗？最近的一项研究证实并非如此。

1)主要结果是造影剂肾病，其诊断标准为肌酐水平在 CT 后 48~72 小时内增加 25% 或 44.2 μmol/L。

2)研究人员发现，与生理盐水组相比，NAC 并没有减少造影剂肾病发生率(每组约 7%)。

3)一个重要的发现是：在急诊科接受 1 升以下静脉液体患者的造影剂肾病发生率是 13%，而接受 1 升以上液体的则为 3%。

3.结论

1)急诊 CT 后可造影剂导致的急性肾损伤发生；

2)NAC 并不比生理盐水更有效；

3)给予超过 1 升的生理盐水将显著降低患造影剂肾病的风险。

参考文献：

McDonald JS, et al. Frequency of acute kidney injury following intravenous contrast medium administration: a systematic reviews and meta-analysis[J]. Radiology, 2013; 267(1): 119-128.

Traub SJ, et al. N-acetylcysteine plus intravenous fluids versus intravenous fluids alone to prevent contrast-induced nephropathy in emergency computed tomography[J]. Ann Emerg Med, 2013; 62 (5): 511-520.

作者：Bryan Hayes

肾脏

胃肠病
Gastroenterology

139. Diarrheal Disease Outbreak in the US

1. General Information:

As of July 30th, 2013, there have been 378 cases of Cyclospora infection from multiple states in the US. Cyclospora is most common in tropical and sub-tropical regions, and is spread via fecal-oral route. While the cause of the most recent outbreak is unknown, outbreaks in the US are generally foodborne.

2. Clinical Presentation:

1) Symptoms usually begin 7 days after exposure.

2) Watery diarrhea, cramping, bloating, nausea, fatigue, increased gas, vomiting, low grade temperature.

3) Can persist several weeks to >1 month.

3. Diagnosis:

Concentrated Stool Ova and Parasites—viewed under modified acid fast or fluorescence microscopy (labs can submit photos to the CDC for "telediagnosis")

4. Treatment:

1) TMP-SMX DS one tab po bid x 7 – 10 days.

2) No effective alternate for failed treatment or sulfa allergy.

3) Most will recover without treatment but S/S can persist for weeks to months.

5. Bottom Line

Consider Cyclospora as a cause of prolonged diarrheal illness, treat with TMP-SMX.

Author: Andrea Tenner

139. 美国流行性腹泻

1.一般资料

截至 2013 年 7 月 30 日，在美国的多个州已经发生 378 例环孢子虫感染。环孢子虫最常见于热带和亚热带地区，通过粪－口途径传播。虽然最近的爆发原因未知，但在美国的爆发流行一般都是食源性的。

2.临床表现

1）通常在接触第 7 天后开始出现症状。

2）水样腹泻，腹部绞痛，腹胀，恶心，疲劳，排气增加，呕吐，低烧。

3）可以持续几个星期到 >1 个月。

3.诊断

粪便找虫卵和寄生虫：可在改良的抗酸性或荧光显微镜下观看到（实验室可以将照片送到疾病预防控制中心做"远程诊断"）。

4.治疗方法复方

1）增效磺胺，口服，一次一片，一天两次，连续服药 7～10 天。

2）对于治疗无效或磺胺过敏者，没有有效的替代药物。

3）即使不治疗，大多数人也会痊愈，但症状和体征可以持续几个星期到几个月。

5.要点

对长期的腹泻性疾病，要考虑孢子虫的原因，治疗用 TMP-SMX。

参考文献：

www.cdc.gov/parasites/cyclosporiasis/outbreaks/investigations－2013.html

作者：Andrea Tenner

胃
肠
病

140. Upper GI Bleeding

1. What findings accurately predict UGI bleeding?

History of prior UGI bleed (likelihood ratio of >6), black stools or melena, Epigastric pain (likelihood ratio of 2.5), Detection of melena on rectal exam (likelihood ratio of 25), BUN: creatinine ratio >30.

2. What findings predict severe UGI bleeding?

Require emergent endoscopy, transfusion, emergent IR or surgical intervention, H/o cirrhosis, malignancy, or syncope, Unstable vital signs/shock (SBP < 100, HR > 100), Hgb < 84, BUN > 90.

3. Treatment of severe bleeding

1) Blood transfusion (consider massive transfusion protocol).

2) Secure airway (consider ketamine).

3) Medications: PPI (although no evidence for survival benefit); If suspect variceal bleeding: Octreotide (best evidence is for decreased transfusion requirement); Antibiotics (3rd generation cephalosporin or quinolone).

4) Rally the troops (GI, IR, Surgery)!

5) Balloon tamponade device.

4. Risk stratification for relatively minor UGI bleed

Glasgow-Blatchford bleeding score (GBS).

(1) http: //www. mdcalc. com/glasgow-blatchford-bleeding-score-gbs/

(2) Questions: BUN, Hgb, sex, h/o CHF or hepatic disease, syncope, VS, presence of melena.

(3) Score is useful only when zero (no deaths or subsequent interventions required).

(4) Does NOT require NG lavage.

5. BOTTOM LINE

1) Best predictors of UGI bleeding are melena on rectal exam and BUN: creatinine ratio >30.

2) Treat severe bleeding aggressively, with transfusion, early activation of consultants, and placement of balloon tamponade device for refractory variceal bleeding.

美
国
急
诊
临
床
必
知
200
招

3)Some patients with minor UGI bleeding can go home! Consider using a scoring system such as the GBS.

4)It's OK to put NG tubes in patients with varices, but overall NG tubes are not all that helpful.

Authors: Mike Winters & Victoria Romaniuk

140. 上消化道出血

1. 如何准确地诊断上消化道出血？

上消化道出血病史（似然比 LR >6），黑便或柏油便，胃区痛（LR 2.5），肛门指检时有柏油便（LR = 25），尿素氮：肌酐比值大于 30。

2. 如何判断严重上消化道出血？

需要紧急内窥镜、输血、紧急放射介入或手术的患者，有肝硬化、肿瘤、晕厥病史，生命体征不稳定/休克（收缩压低于 100 mmHg，心率高于 100 次/分），血红蛋白低于 8.4 g，尿素氮高于 90 mmol/L。

3. 大出血的治疗：

1）输血（考虑大输血方案）。

2）保护气道（考虑用氯胺酮）。

3）药物：质子泵抑制药（虽然尚无有益于生存的证据）；如怀疑有静脉曲张出血，要用奥曲肽（最有力的证据是减少对输血的需求）；抗菌素（3 代头孢或喹诺酮类）。

4）召集队伍（胃肠科，放射介入，外科医生）。

5）气囊填塞设备。

4. 相对小量上消化道出血的危险因素分析

Glasgow-Blatchford 出血分数（GBS）：

（1）GBS 分数相关内容可在相应网站获取。

（2）计分项目：尿素氮、血红蛋白、性别、心力衰竭、肝病、晕厥、生命体征、柏油便。

（3）分数只有为零时才有意义（没有死亡并不需要介入治疗）。

（4）不需要放置胃管灌洗。

5. 要点

1）判断上消化道出血的最好的指标是肛检有柏油便和尿素氮：肌酐 >30。

2）积极治疗大出血，包括输血、早期会诊和对顽固性曲张出血使用气囊填塞。

3）有些小量出血的患者可以回家，也可参考使用 GBS 评分系统。

4）有静脉曲张的患者可以放胃管，但总的来讲帮助不大。

美
国
急
诊
临
床
必
知
200
招

参考文献:

Srygley FD, Gerardo CJ, Tran T, Fisher DA. Does This Patient Have a Severe Upper Gastrointestinal Bleed? JAMA. 2012; 307(10): 1072 – 1079.

Ali H, Lang E, Barkan A. Emergency department risk stratification in upper gastrointestinal bleeding. CJEM. 2012 Jan; 14(1): 45 – 49.

作者: **Mike Winters & Victoria Romaniuk**

胃
肠
病

内分泌
Endocrinology

141. Glycemic Control and Cardiovascular Risk

1. Tight glycemic control (HbA1C < 7%) has previously been recommended in CAD based on data from the United Kingdom Prospective Diabetes Study (UKPDS)

2. A recent study evaluated the relationship between glycemic control, cardiovascular disease (CVD) risk, and all-cause mortality.

3. Patients with a mean HbA1C 7% − 7.4% were compared to those with mean HbA1C < 6%; tight glycemic control had a 68% increased risk of CVD hospitalization

4. HbA1C > 8.5% also had significantly higher risk.

5. CVD risk and all-cause mortality is greater with both aggressive and lax glycemic control and the optimal reference range may lie between 7% − 7.4%

Author: Semhar Tewelde

141. 血糖控制和心血管危险因素

1. 根据英国前瞻性糖尿病研究(UKPDS)的结果,加拿大糖尿病协会(CAD)已建议要严格控制血糖[糖化血红蛋白(HbA1c) <7%]。

2. 最近的一项研究评估了血糖控制、心血管疾病(CVD)的风险以及各种原因的死亡之间的关系。

3. 对平均 HbAlc 7% ~7.4% 和 <6% 的患者进行比较,发现过于严格控制血糖使心血管疾病患者住院的风险增加68%。

4. HbAlc >8.5% 也明显增加了这一风险。

5. 过于严格控制或血糖控制不佳都大幅度增加了心血管疾病的风险和全因死亡率。最理想的糖化血红蛋白参考范围可能是介于7% ~7.4% 之间。

参考文献:

Nichols G, Joshua-Gotlib S, Parasuraman. Glycemic Control and Risk of Cardiovascular Disease Hospitalization and All-Cause Mortality. JACC. 2013; 62: 2; 121 – 127.

作者:**Semhar Tewelde**

内
分
泌

血液和肿瘤病
Hematology and Oncology

142. Immune Thrombocytopenia Purpura (ITP)

1. Keep Immune Thrombocytopenic Purpura (ITP) in your differential for patients with thrombocytopenia and evidence of bleeding. Although ITP has classically been described in children, it can occur in adults; especially between 3rd-4th decade.

2. Thrombocytopenia leads to the extravasation of blood from capillaries, leading to skin bruising, mucus membrane petechial bleeding, and intracranial hemorrhage.

3. ITP occurs from production of auto-antibodies which bind to circulating platelets. This leads to irreversible uptake by macrophages in the spleen. Causes of antibody production include:

1) Medication exposure.

2) Infection (usually viral), including HIV and hepatitis.

3) Immune disorders (e. g. , lupus).

4) Pregnancy.

5) Idiopathic.

4. Suspect ITP in patients with isolated thrombocytopenia on a CBC without other blood-line abnormalities. Abnormality in other blood-line warrants consideration of another diagnosis (e. g. , leukemia).

5. ITP cannot be cured; treatments include:

1) Steroid to suppress antibody production (first-line therapy).

2) Intravenous immunoglobulin (IVIG).

3) IV Rho immunoglobulin (for Rh + patients only).

4) Rituximab +/ − dexamethasone.

5) Splenectomy (rare cases of massive hemorrhage refractory to pharmacologic treatment).

Author: Haney Mallemat

142. 免疫性血小板减少性紫癜(ITP)

1. 对有血小板减少和出血证据的患者,应考虑可能为免疫性血小板减少性紫癜(ITP)。尽管传统认为 ITP 仅在儿童间发病,但它可以发生在成人,尤其是30～40岁年龄段。

2. 血小板减少导致血液从毛细血管渗出,出现皮肤青紫、黏膜瘀点状出血和颅内出血。

3. ITP 的发生是由于循环中血小板与自身抗体的结合导致脾巨噬细胞对血小板的不可逆转破坏。抗体产生的原因包括:

1)药物;

2)感染(通常是病毒感染),包括艾滋病毒和肝炎;

3)免疫紊乱(如红斑狼疮);

4)怀孕;

5)特发性。

4. 对于全血细胞计数显示血小板减少但没有其他血象异常的患者要怀疑ITP。如有其他血象异常值得考虑另外的诊断(如白血病)。

5. ITP 不能治愈,治疗方法包括:

1)用激素抑制抗体的产生(一线治疗);

2)静脉注射免疫球蛋白(IVIG);

3)静脉用 Rho 免疫球蛋白[只限于 RH(＋)患者];

4)利妥昔单抗单用或合用地塞米松;

5)脾切除术(罕见的对药物治疗无效的大出血病例)。

作者: Haney Mallemat

血液和肿瘤病

335

143. Thalassemia

1. A genetic autosomal recessive blood disorders that result from a defect in either the alpha (α) or Beta (β) globin chain in the hemoglobin molecule.

2. Most common in people from a Mediterranean origin.

3. Three types depending on the affected globin chain, α, β, or Delta (δ).

4. Presents as hemolytic anemia with hepato-splenomegaly.

5. Can present as mild anemia and may be misdiagnosed as iron deficiency anemia.

6. Diagnosis is made through studies such as bone marrow examination, hemoglobin electrophoresis, and iron studies.

7. The disease can cause hemochromatosis, which may be worsened by repeated blood transfusions.

8. Hemochromatosis damages multiple organs including the Liver, spleen, endocrine glands and the heart causing cardiomyopathy and consequently heart failure.

9. Severe thalassemia usually requires blood transfusion on regular basis (first measure effective in prolonging life).

10. Treatment of trait cases is symptomatic with analgesics, anti-inflammatory(steroids or NSAIDs).

11. The introduction of chelating agents capable of removing excessive iron from the body has dramatically increased life expectancy.

12. Deferasirox (Exjade) was approved by the FDA in January 2013 for treatment of chronic iron overload caused by nontransfusion-dependent thalassemia.

Author: Walid Hammad

143. 地中海贫血

1. 地中海贫血是因血红蛋白分子球蛋白 α 或 β 链上有缺陷而导致的一种常染色体隐性遗传的血液疾病。

2. 在地中海人群中最常见。

3. 根据受影响的球蛋白链不同可分成 α，β，δ 3 种。

4. 其表现为伴有肝脾肿大的溶血性贫血。

5. 有时会表现为轻度贫血，容易误诊为缺铁性贫血。

6. 主要通过骨髓活检、血红蛋白电泳和血清铁检查确诊。

7. 该病可导致血色素沉着症，反复输血可以使病情恶化。

8. 血色素沉着症可引发多脏器(肝脏、脾脏、内分泌腺和心脏)损伤，并导致心肌肥厚和心力衰竭。

9. 严重的地中海贫血通常需要有规律的输血(延长生命的首要办法)。

10. 对于轻型的患者主要是对症治疗、止痛、消炎(激素或非激素类抗炎药)。

11. 能够从体内排出过多铁的螯合剂可显著延长患者生命。

12. 地拉罗斯(恩瑞格)在 2013 年 1 月被美国 FDA 批准可以用来治疗地中海贫血患者中非输血性慢性铁超负荷的治疗。

参考文献：

Delvecchio M，Cavallo L. Growth and endocrine function in thalassemia major in childhood and adolescence. J Endocrinol Invest. Jan 2010；33(1)：61 – 68

Claude Owen Burdick. "Separating Thalassemia Trait and Iron Deficiency by Simple Inspection". American Society for Clinical Pathology.

http：//ajcp. ascpjournals. org/content/131/3/444. short

作者：Walid Hammad

血液和肿瘤病

337

眼科疾病
Ophthalmology

144. Treating conjunctivitis with antibiotics

1. Children frequently present with "pink eye" to the ED. When they do, parents often expect antibiotics. How many of these kids actually need them? Previous studies have shown approximately 54% of acute conjunctivitis was bacterial, but antibiotics were prescribed in 80 – 95% of cases.

2. A prospective study in a suburban children's hospital published in 2007, showed that 87% of the cases during the study period were bacterial. The most common type of bacteria was nontypeable H. influenza followed by S. pneumoniae.

3. Topical antibiotic treatment has been shown to improve remission rates by 6 – 10 days.

Author: Jennifer Guyther

144. 结膜炎的抗生素治疗

1. 儿童经常因"红眼病"到急诊科就诊,当他们来时,父母总是盼望能给予抗生素治疗。这些孩子中有多少人真正需要抗生素呢?以往的研究表明,约54%的急性结膜炎是细菌性的,但有80%~95%的患者接受了抗生素治疗。

2. 在2007年发表的来自于一个郊区儿童医院的前瞻性研究结果表明:在研究期间,87%的患者为细菌性结膜炎。最常见的细菌为不可分型的流感嗜血杆菌,其次是肺炎链球菌。

3. 外用抗生素治疗已被证明能提前6~10天提高缓解率。

参考文献:

Patel et al. Clinical Features of Bacterial Conjunctivitis in Children. Academic Emergency Medicine 2007;14:1-5.

作者:Jennifer Guyther

眼科疾病

妇产科
Gynecology and Obstetrics

145. Simple tips for managing the critically-Ⅲ pregnant patient

1. The pregnant patient normally has increased cardiac output and minute ventilation by the third trimester. Despite this increase, however, these patients have little cardiopulmonary reserve should they become critically-ill.

2. Remember the mnemonic T. O. L. D. D. for simple tips that should be done for the pregnant patient who presents critically-ill or with the potential for critical illness:

1) Tilt: The supine-hypotension syndrome occurs after the 20th week of pregnancy as the gravid uterus compresses the IVC and aorta, reducing cardiac output by up to 30%. Placing a 30-degree right hip-wedge under the patient will relieve this obstruction.

2) Oxygen: the growing uterus pushes up on the base of the lungs reducing the functional residual capacity meaning there is less oxygen reserve and rapid oxygen desaturations. Supplemental oxygen may increase the patient's reserve.

3) Lines: The circulatory system reserve is reduced, so early and large bore venous access is important. Remember that lines should be placed above the diaphragm because the enlarging uterus compresses pelvic veins, reducing venous return to the heart.

4) Dates: Rapidly determine the gestational age of the fetus as 24 weeks is a critical date to remember (e. g. , increased risk of supine-hypotension syndrome, fetal viability, etc.)

5) Delivery: Call labor and delivery early on, not only for the consultation, but also for the fetal monitoring that this service provides.

Author: Haney Mallemat

145.治疗病危怀孕患者的简单技巧

1.孕妇通常在孕晚期出现心输出量和每分钟通气量增加,尽管这样,她们一旦患重病,其心肺功能储备就会不够。

2.在治疗病危或有发生病危倾向的孕妇时,要记住这个简单的口诀 T. O. L. D. D.:

1)倾斜(tilt)。仰卧位低血压综合征通常出现在怀孕 20 周后,由于妊娠子宫压迫下腔静脉和主动脉,心输出量减少高达 30% 。在孕妇右髋下方放置一个 30° 的楔形物可缓解这一压迫。

2)氧气(oxygen)。不断增大的子宫将肺底部向上推移,降低肺部功能残气量,使氧气储备减少和氧饱和度下降加快。补充氧气可增加患者的氧储备。

3)静脉通路(lines)。由于循环系统储备减少,所以早期建立大静脉通路是非常重要的。请记住静脉通路应放在横膈膜以上的位置,因为扩大的子宫压迫盆腔静脉,减少下肢静脉血回流到心脏。

4)日期(dates)。迅速确定胎龄,因为 24 周的胎龄是一个关键(例如,仰卧位低血压综合征的风险增加,胎儿已有生存能力等)。

5)分娩(delivery)。尽早联系产科,不仅仅是为了会诊,同时也要提供胎儿监护。

作者:Haney Mallemat

皮肤病
Dermatology

146. Is that rash a mess? Maybe it's DRESS.

1. DRESS (Drug Reaction with Eosinophilia and Systemic Symptoms) or DIHS (Drug-Induced Hypersensitivity Syndrome) is a potentially life-threatening adverse drug-reaction.

2. Incidence is 1/1, 000 to 1/10, 00 drug exposures. It occurs 2 – 6 weeks after the drug is first introduced, distinguishing it from other adverse drug-reactions which typically occur sooner.

3. The syndrome classically includes:

1) Severe skin eruptions (typically morbilliform or erythrodermic eruptions).

2) Hematologic abnormalities (eosinophilia or atypical lymphocytosis).

3) Organ involvement; e. g. , hepatic (most common), pneumonitis, renal failure, etc.

4) Fevers.

5) Arthralgia.

6) Lymphadenopathy.

4. The most commonly implicated drugs are anticonvulsants (e. g. , carbamazepine, phenobarbital, and phenytoin), sulfonamides, and allopurinol.

5. Recovery is typically complete after discontinuing the offending drug; systemic steroids may promote resolution of the illness.

Author: Haney Mallemat

美
国
急
诊
临
床
必
知
200
招

146. 伴有嗜酸性粒细胞增多和全身症状的药物不良反应

1. DRESS(伴有嗜酸性粒细胞增多和全身症状的药物不良反应)或 DIHS(药物超敏反应综合征)是一种潜在的可致命的药物不良反应。

2. 在药物接触人群中的发生率为 1/1000 ~ 1/10000。有别于其他药物不良反应，DRESS 一般在首次接触药物 2 ~ 6 周后出现，

3. 该综合征的典型表现包括：

1)严重的皮疹(典型麻疹样或红皮病)；

2)血液学异常(嗜酸性粒细胞增多或非特异性淋巴细胞增多症)；

3)器官损伤：肝脏(最常见)、肺炎、肾衰等；

4)发热；

5)关节痛；

6)淋巴结肿大。

4. 最常见的药物有：抗癫痫药(卡马西平、苯巴比妥、苯妥英钠)，磺胺类药和别嘌呤醇。

5. 在停药后可完全恢复，全身用激素对疾病的恢复有帮助。

参考文献：

Cacoub P. et al. The DRESS syndrome：a literature review. Am J Med 2011 Jul；124(7)：588 – 597.

作者：**Haney Mallemat**

皮肤病

国际区域性疾病
Global Health

147. Typhoid Fever

1. General information

1) Salmonella typhi-transmission through fecal-oral, contaminated food, human carriers.

2) Most cases in the US acquired abroad-Africa, Latin American, Asia.

3) Vaccine available-not life-long immunity, need 1 − 2 weeks to take effect.

2. Clinical Presentation:

1) sustained high fever (103 − 104).

2) Faget sign: fever and bradycardia (also seen in yellow fever, atypical pneumonia, tularemia, brucellosis, Colorado tick fever).

3) Abdominal pain, GI bleed/perforation, hepatosplenomegaly, delirium.

4) "Rose spots"-erythematous macular rash over chest and abdomen.

5) Without treatment sx can resolve after 3 − 4 weeks, mortality from secondary infections 12% − 30%.

3. Diagnosis:

1) Pan-culture for S. typhi.

2) Serologic: Widal test (negative for 1st week of symptoms, 7 − 14 days to result).

4. Treatment:

1) Abx: amoxicillin, trimethoprim-sulfamethoxazole, and ciprofloxacin.

2) MDR typhoid: ceftriaxone or Azithromycine 1st line.

5. Bottom Line:

1) Get vaccinated if travelling to endemic areas 1 − 2 weeks before travel.

2) Suspect in travelers to endemic areas with sustained high fevers.

3) Spontaneous resolution does occur but may become carriers without abx.

Author: Walid Hammad

147. 伤寒

1. 一般资料

1) 伤寒沙门氏菌通过粪 - 口途径、受污染的食物和人携带者传播。

2) 美国的大多数病例都是在国外获得 - 非洲、拉丁美洲、亚洲。

3) 注射疫苗后需要 1~2 周才能生效,但不是终身免疫。

2. 临床表现

1) 持续高热(39.4℃~40℃)。

2) 费格特(Faget)征:发热和心动过缓(也可见于黄热病、非典型性肺炎、土拉菌病、布氏杆菌病、科罗拉多蜱热)。

3) 腹痛、消化道出血/穿孔、肝脾肿大、神志昏迷。

4) "玫瑰斑":胸部和腹部红斑疹。

5) 如果不进行治疗,症状可在 3~4 周后消失,因继发感染而死亡的约占12%~30%。

3. 诊断

1) 伤寒沙门氏菌的全部培养。

2) 血清:肥达氏试验(第一周内指标可呈阴性,7~14 天才能出结果)

4. 治疗方法

1) 抗生素:阿莫西林,复方新诺明,环丙沙星。

2) 多药物耐药(MDR)伤寒:一线药为头孢曲松,阿奇霉素。

5. 要点

1) 要在前往流行地区前 1~2 周接种疫苗。

2) 如发现到流行地区的旅客有持续高热,要怀疑此病。

3) 此病可自愈,但如果没有便用抗生素有成为携带者的可能。

作者:Walid Hammad

国际区域性疾病

148. Relapsing fever

1. Causative organism: members of the genus Borrelia.

2. 1) Louse Borne Relapsing Fever (LBRF)

Human body louse (Pediculushumanus).

Associated with sporadic outbreaks especially in areas with large refugee populations.

2) Tick Borne Relapsing Fever (TBRF)

Soft ticks of the genus Ornithodoros.

Typically found in higher elevations of the western United States as well as the central plateau region of Mexico, Central and South America and Africa.

3. Clinical Presentation

1) Symptoms develop 3 to 18 days after infection.

2) Onset is abrupt and may include fever, malaise, headache, arthralgias, nausea and vomiting and cough.

3) The first febrile episode lasts 3 to 6 days and then recurrences may occur after 7 to 10 days.

4. Diagnosis

1) Definitive diagnosis: visualization of spirochetes on peripheral blood smear.

2) May also see leukocytosis, anemia and/or thrombocytopenia, elevation of liver function tests.

3) Erythrocyte rosette formation may be present.

5. Treatment

1) Antibiotics recommended for treatment include penicillin, doxycycline and erythromycin.

2) Jarisch-Herxheimer reaction common after treatment. This can be life threatening and all patients undergoing treatment should be closely monitored.

Author: Gentry Wilkerson

148. 回归热

1.致病菌：莱姆菌系。

2.1)虱子传播的回归热(LBRF)：

人体虱(Pediculushumanus)；

与散在的爆发有关，尤其在难民多的地区。

2)蜱传播的回归热(TBRF)：

软蜱族，纯绿蜱属（Ornithodoros）；

主要分布在美国西部的高海拔地带和墨西哥、中南美及非洲的中心平原地带。

3.临床表现

1)症状在感染后3~18天出现。

2)症状常突然出现，包括发热、乏力、头疼、关节痛、恶心、呕吐、咳嗽。

3)第一次发热期持续3~6天，常在7~10天后复发。

4.诊断

1)确诊：外周血涂片中查到螺旋体。

2)可出现白细胞增高、贫血、血小板低、肝功能异常。

3)红细胞花环形成。

5.治疗

1)抗生素：青霉素、四环素、红霉素。

2)治疗后常会出现Jarisch-Herxheimer反应，可危及生命，因此要对治疗中的患者进行密切观察。

参考文献：

Centers for Disease Control and Prevention CDC. Tickborne relapsing fever in a mother and newborn child—Colorado, 2011. MMWR Morb Mortal Wkly Rep. 2012；61(10)：174-176.

Larsson C, Andersson M, Bergström S. Current issues in relapsing fever. CurrOpin Infect Dis. 2009；22(5)：443-449.

作者：Gentry Wilkerson

国际区域性疾病

149. Cholera

1. Diagnosis should be considered in any individual over 5 years old with severe dehydration from diarrhea, regardless of exposure to an endemic area, and any patient over 2 years old with watery diarrhea in an endemic area.

2. Patients with severe cholera can stool as much as 1 L an hour. Replacing fluids is the most important part of treatment with oral rehydration being used as soon as possible.

3. Oral rehydrationtherapy provides better potassium, carbohydrate, and bicarbonate replacement than most IV fluid solutions.

4. Antibiotics will also decrease volume and duration of stooling but are only recommended in moderate to severe illness.

5. Antiemetics are not useful because they can make patients sleepy and will reduce their ability to rehydrate orally.

6. Antimotility medications will prolong the duration of illness.

Author: Jenny Reifel Saltzberg

149. 霍乱

1. 对任何一个 5 岁以上由于腹泻造成的严重脱水的患者，不论是否到过霍乱流行区，都要考虑霍乱的可能性。在霍乱流行区，任何一个 2 岁以上有稀水便的患者，都要考虑霍乱。

2. 严重霍乱患者可每小时排稀便 1 升以上，因此，补水是最重要的治疗手段。口服补液开始得越早越好。

3. 与静脉输液相比，口服补液可提供更合理的钾、氯和碳酸钠成分。

4. 抗生素会减少患者排便量和缩短腹泻时间，但只推荐对中重度患者使用。

5. 止呕药会使患者感觉疲倦和嗜睡，达不到口服补液的效果，不推荐临床使用。

6. 止泻药会延长疾病的时间。

参考文献：

Harris JB, LaRocque RC, Qadri F, Ryan ET, Calderwood SB. Cholera. Lancet. 2012 Jun 30；379(9835)：2466 – 2476.

国际区域性疾病

150. Hantavirus (Sin Nombre Virus)

1. General Information

1)Organism: Bunyaviridae virus.

2)Infection occurs through inhalation of aerosols contaminated with rodent urine or feces.

3)Animal reservoir-rodents.

4)Seen more commonly in the southwestern United States.

5)Death occurs from decreased cardiac output and circulatory failure.

2. Clinical Presentation

1)Initial symptoms are nonspecific: fever, malaise, and myalgia; but can progress to fulminant ARDS-like picture in previously health young patients.

2)Two syndromes

(1)Hantapulmonary syndrome (HPS)

Pulmonary symptoms follow the initial prodrome and include tachypnea, hypoxia, and respiratory distress; pulmonary involvement can rapidly progress to ARDS.

(2)Hemorrhagic Fever with Renal Syndrome (HFRS)

Hematologic dysfunction with hemorrhage, retroperitoneal fluids, renal failure, shock.

3. Diagnosis

1)The diagnosis must initially be made clinically.

2)Lab tests may reveal nonspecific findings of thrombocytopenia, hemoconcentration, and renal failure.

3)Chest film will demonstrate bilateral interstitial infiltrates.

4)PCR can demonstrate hantavirus-specific antibodies.

4. Treatment

There is no specific therapy for hantavirus infection; Treatment is primarily supportive, with attention to respiratory status and oxygenation.

Author: Andi Tenner

150. 汉坦病毒

1. 一般资料

1) 致病菌：布尼亚病毒（Bunyaviridae）。

2) 感染途径：吸入啮齿动物尿或粪便污染的空气微粒。

3) 动物宿主：啮齿动物。

4) 常见于美国的西南部。

5) 死因多为心输出量下降和循环衰竭。

2. 临床表现

1) 最初症状都不特异：发烧、乏力和肌肉酸痛；但在健康的年轻患者中可能恶化成成人呼吸窘迫综合征（ARDS）。

2) 两类症状

（1）汉坦病毒肺综合征（HPS）

表现包括：心动过速、缺氧和呼吸困难；会很快转化为 ARDS。

（2）出血热伴肾脏损伤（HFRS）

血液系统的功能紊乱可导致出血、腹膜后积液、肾功能衰竭和休克。

3. 诊断

1) 最初诊断要根据临床表现确定。

2) 实验室检查可发现非特异的血小板减少、血液浓缩和肾功能衰竭。

3) 胸片显示双侧间质浸润影。

4) PCR 显示汉坦病毒特异性抗体。

4. 治疗

对汉坦病毒感染没有特异性的治疗方案，主要是以保持通气和吸氧为主的呼吸支持疗法。

参考文献：

Center for Disease Control. (2012). Hantavirus. Retrieved September 3, 2012, from

Berger, S. A., Calisher, C. H., and Keystone, J. H., (2003). Exotic Viral Disease：A Global Guide. Hamilton, Ontario：BC Decker.

作者：**Andi Tenner**

国际区域性疾病

151. Dengue

1. Dengue is the most rapidly expanding mosquito-borne virus with an increasing incidence and geographical area. The disease is most commonly found in the tropics, but there are occasional outbreaks in other places including Texas and Hawaii.

2. Dengue has 3 phases.

1) The febrile phase lasts 2 – 7 days and is similar to viral syndrome: high fever with nausea and vomiting. There may also be petechiae which can be induced by the application of a tourniquet.

2) The critical phase occurs after defervescence and lasts only 24 – 48 hours. It is marked by increased capillary permeability and can lead to severe pulmonary edema, shock, and multisystem organ failure.

3) The recovery phase is marked by hemodynamic improvement. Some patients have a rash described as "isles of white in a sea of red." Some patients will develop bradycardia.

3. Most patients have a self-limited form of the illness that is not severe, and consists of symptoms seen in the febrile phase. The patients that develop severe dengue can have markers in the febrile phase that are associated with organ dysfunction, GI bleeding, and increased capillary permeability. Other concerning symptoms early are abdominal tenderness or persistent vomiting.

4. Treatment is supportive, mostly consisting of IV fluids, which is very effective when started early in the patient's illness.

Author: Andi Tenner

151. 登革热

1. 登革热是由蚊子导致的目前传播最快的病毒性疾病, 它的发病率和流行区域都有增加的趋势。登革热在热带最常见, 偶尔也可以在其他地区暴发, 如德克萨斯和夏威夷。

2. 登革热有三期

1) 发热期, 多持续 2~7 天, 与普通病毒感染症状相似: 伴有恶心和呕吐的高热。可出现出血点, 尤其在用止血带的地方。

2) 极期在退热后开始, 可持续 24~48 小时, 主要表现为由毛细血管通透性增加导致的严重肺水肿、休克和多脏器功能衰竭。

3) 恢复期的标志为血液动力学的改善。有些患者会出现"皮岛"样的皮疹。

3. 绝大多数只有发热期症状的患者均可自愈, 重症患者在发热期就会出现器官功能紊乱、消化道出血和毛细血管通透性增加。其他早期的症状包括腹部触痛及顽固性呕吐。

4. 治疗以支持和辅助治疗为主, 主要是静脉补液, 在疾病的早期开始补液是一种非常有效的治疗措施。

参考文献:

Dengue: guidelines for diagnosis, treatment, prevention and control-New Edition. (2009) World Health Organization.

Chen LH, Wilson ME. Dengue and chikungunya in travelers: recent updates. Curr Opin Infect Dis 2012 Oct; 25(5): 523 – 529.

作者: **Andi Tenner**

国际区域性疾病

152. Human African trypanosomiasis?

1. Human African trypanosomiasis (HAT) , also known as " sleeping sickness"

2. A parasitic disease transmitted by the bite of the 'Glossina' insect (tsetse fly.)

3. The disease is most prevalent in rural areas of Africa. Untreated, it is usually fatal. Infection with the genus Trypanosoma brucei gambiense may lead to chronic asymptomatic illness.

4. Travelers to endemic areas in Africa are risk becoming infected.

5. Symptoms resemble a viral illness; headaches, fever, weakness, pain in the joints, and stiffness. The parasite is able to crosses the blood-brain barrier and causes neurological symptoms, mainly psychiatric disorders, seizures, coma and ultimately death.

6. Diagnosis is by serological tests (Card Agglutination Trypanosomiasis Test or CATT). Confirmation of infection requires the performance of parasitological tests to demonstrate the presence of trypanosomes in the patient.

7. Treatment: four drugs are registered for the treatment of HAT: pentamidine, suramin, melarsoprol and eflornithine.

Author

152. 非洲人类锥虫病

1. 非洲人类锥虫病，又称嗜睡病。

2. 这是一种由"舌蝇"（采采蝇）传播的寄生虫病。

3. 此病在非洲边远地区最为流行，如不治疗，常危及生命。由布氏冈比亚锥虫所致的感染常会演变成慢性无症状疾病。

4. 到非洲流行区的旅游者有被感染的风险。

5. 症状与病毒感染相似：头痛、发烧、乏力，关节痛和关节僵硬。寄生虫可以通过血脑屏障引发神经系统异常，如精神紊乱、癫痫、昏迷，最终导致死亡。

6. 诊断主要通过血清学检查（锥虫凝集卡试验，CATT），确诊需要在患者体内检出锥虫。

7. 治疗：苏拉明、喷他脒、硫胂密胺和依氟鸟氨酸均可用来治疗非洲人类锥虫病。

参考文献：

World Health Organization. (2010). Working to overcome the global impact of neglected tropical diseases. First WHO report on neglected tropical diseases. Available：http：//whqlibdoc. who. int/publications/2010/9789241564090_eng. pdf. Last accessed 12/17/2012

作者：

国际区域性疾病

153. Leptospirosis

1. General Information:

1)Leptospirosis is a tropical infectious disease that is also endemic in the US. (Estimated 16% seroprevalence in inner city Baltimore!)

2)The spirochete is spread through animal urine and can survive in water or soil for weeks.

3)Risk factors: rural exposure to animal urine (farming, adventure sports) or urban exposure to rat urine.

4)Infection is acquired through breaks in the skin or mucus membranes

5)Outbreaks are often seen following rain or floods.

2. Clinical Presentation:

1)Non-specific febrile illness (usually not diagnosed in these cases)

2)If untreated, 5% – 10% progress to jaundice, renal failure, thrombocytopenia, hemorrhage, and respiratory failure.

3. Diagnosis:

1)Primarily based on clinical presentation and history.

2)Paired serum sent to CDC (the acute serum sample should be drawn in the ED).

4. Treatment:

Doxycycline, Ceftriaxone and Penicillin are all effective.

5. Bottom Line:

Consider and treat for Leptospirosis in patients with possible exposure animal urine (especially after a flood) who present in extremis with renal failure, jaundice, and thrombocytopenia.

Author: Andi Tenner

153. 钩端螺旋体病

简述：

钩端螺旋体病是一种热带感染性疾病，在美国也有流行（在巴尔的摩内城区约有 16% 的居民血清呈阳性）。

钩端螺旋体通过动物尿液传播，在水或土壤中可存活几周。

1. 致病因素

1）与动物尿有直接接触（耕作，探险运动）或城市内接触老鼠尿液。

2）通过损伤的皮肤或黏膜感染。

3）雨后或洪水后常出现暴发流行。

2. 临床表现

1）非特异性发热性疾病（在这一阶段常漏诊）。

2）如不治疗，5% ~10% 的患者会出现黄疸、肾功能衰竭、血小板减少、出血和呼吸衰竭。

3. 诊断

1）主要根据病史和临床表现来判断。

2）将血清送到 CDC（急性期的血清应在急诊科采取）。

4. 治疗

四环素、头孢曲松和青霉素都有效。

5. 要点

对与动物尿有接触后（尤其在洪水后）出现肾功衰竭、黄疸和血小板减少的患者要考虑钩端螺旋体病。

参考文献：

Childs JE, Schwartz BS, Ksiazek TG, et al. Risk Factors Associated with Antibodies to Leptospires in Inner-city Residents of Baltimore：A Protective Role for Cats. Am J Public Health. 1992；82：597 – 599.

Leung J, Schiffer J. Feverish, Jaundiced. Am J Med. 2009；122：129 – 131.

Center for Disease Control. (2012) Leptospirosis. Retrieved January 1, 2013 from

作者：**Andi Tenner**

国际区域性疾病

154. Malaria (一)

1. General information:

1)Organism: 5 Plasmodium species (P. falciparum, P. vivax, P. ovale, P. malari-ae, P. knowlesi)

2)P. falciparum is responsible for most severe disease.

3)P. vivax and P. ovale are responsible for recrudescent disease.

4)Transmission via the female Anopheles mosquito, which bites at night or in the early morning.

5)Endemic in Asia, Africa, Central America, and South America

2. Clinical presentation:

1)Initially, the patient presents with an acute febrile illness: fever, chills, head-ache, nausea, lethargy, and upper respiratory symptoms.

2)Infection with P. falciparum can further progress to severe organ dysfunction.

3)The disease course is unpredictable in the non-immune individual.

3. Diagnosis:

1)Thick and thin peripheral blood smears demonstrating organism.

2)Thick smear-confirms Plasmodium parasites.

3)Thin smear-allows speciation of Plasmodium parasites.

4)Hyperparasitemia is associated with increased mortality.

4. Treatment:

1)P. falciparum or species unidentified.

2)For severe malaria, IV quinine (quinidine if quinine not available).

3)IV artesunate is available from the CDC as a quinidine/quinine alternative.

4)DO NOT USE Chloroquine for severe malaria.

5)Patients with evidence of complicated malaria (>3% parasitemia, signs of or-gan dysfunction, alterations in mental status) should be admitted to an ICU.

Author: Emilie J. B. Calvello

154. 疟疾(一)

1. 基本信息

1)致病微生物：5 种疟原虫(恶性疟原虫、间日疟原虫、卵形疟原虫、三日疟原虫、诺氏疟原虫)。

2)恶性疟原虫常导致严重的疾病。

3)间日疟原虫和卵形疟原虫常导致疾病复发。

4)传播途径是雌性按蚊叮咬，经常在晚上或凌晨发生。

5)流行区包括亚洲、非洲、中美洲和南美洲。

2. 临床表现

1)患者常以急性发热性疾病就诊：发烧、寒战、头疼、恶心、嗜睡及上呼吸道症状。

2)恶性疟原虫感染可能发展成严重的器官衰竭。

3)对于一个没有免疫力的患者来说，病程是不可预测的。

3. 诊断

1)血液涂片(薄片和厚片)查疟原虫。

2)厚涂片：可证实有疟原虫的存在。

3)薄涂片：可鉴别疟原虫类别。

4)高疟原虫血症与高死亡率密切相关。

4. 治疗

1)恶性疟或不明种类。

2)对重度感染者可静脉注射奎宁，如没有奎宁，可用奎尼丁。

3)作为奎宁和奎尼丁的替代药，可以向 CDC 寻求青蒿琥酯静脉注射。

4)严重的疟疾禁用氯奎。

5)对于有明确复杂疟疾的患者(3% 以上有疟原虫血症、器官衰竭表现及神志改变)要收入重症监护病房。

参考文献：

Center for Disease Control. (2012). Malaria. Retrieved November 9, 2012, from http：//www. cdc. gov/MALARIA

Wattal, C. et al. Infectious disease emergencies in returning travelers：special referece to malaria, dengue and chikungunya. Med Clin North Am. 2012 Nov；96(6)：1225 – 1255.

作者：**Emilie J. B. Calvello**

国际区域性疾病

155. Malaria (二)

1. Case Presentation from our ED

20 y/o presents 3 weeks after emigrating from Senegal with headache and malaise. CT/LP and work up was otherwise negative. Thin smear shows 1 plasmodium falciparum parasite in 7000 RBC.

Appropriate therapy is initiated with malarone (atovoquone and progranuil). 24 hours later the patient represents with worsening headache and fever.

Repeat smear shows 10% parasitemia and massive numbers of parasites

2. Clinical Question: Can parasitemia rise after initiation of treatment?

Answer: Yes.

3. Increase in blood parasite count in falciparum malaria after initiation of treatment (artemisinin derivatives or quinine) is not uncommon.

Increased blood parasite count does not indicated treatment failure if it the parasitemia is LESS THAN 2.5 x the baseline count.

4. Clinical Question: Did this patient have treatment failure with malarone?

Answer: Yes.

The patient's parasitemia rose to 10% after initiation of therapy.

There are increasing case reports of treatment failure in West Africa with Malarone.

5. Bottom Line: A mild increase in blood parasite count after initiation of treatment is not uncommon. Marked increases should indicated treatment failure and the treatment drug should be changed to another class.

Author: Emilie J. B. Calvello

155. 疟疾续(二)

1. 急诊科病例一例:

一位从塞内加尔到美国 3 周的 20 岁的患者,因头痛和乏力就诊。所有的检查包括 CT 和腰椎穿刺都无异常。薄片检查发现在 7000 个红细胞中有一个恶性疟原虫。

患者及时接受了针对性药物马拉隆(阿托喹酮和氯胍)的治疗。24 小时后,患者头痛和发烧症状加重。

重复薄片检查发现 10% 寄生虫血症和大量寄生虫。

2. 问题:治疗开始后会出现寄生虫血症吗?

答案:会的。

3. 恶性疟原虫病在治疗(青蒿素衍生物或奎宁)开始后血中疟原虫数量增加现象是常见的。

如果寄生虫血症不超过基础水平的 2.5 倍,并不代表治疗无效。

4. 问题:这个患者用马拉隆治疗是失败了吗?

答案:是的。

因为患者的寄生虫血症在治疗开始后增加到了 10%。

在西非,用马拉隆治疗失败的病例有增加的趋势。

5. 要点

治疗后血液中寄生虫出现轻微增长并不罕见,大幅度的增加意味着治疗的失败,应考虑换用其他类的药物。

参考文献:

Wurts, N. Et al. Early treatment failure during treatment of Plasmodium falciparum malaria with atovaquone-proquanil in the Repulic of Ivory Coast. Malar J 2012 May;2(11):146.

Silachomroon, U. Et al. Frequency of Early Rising Parasitemia in Falciparum Malaria Treated with Artemisinin Derivatives. Southeast Asian J Trop Med Pub Health 2001 Mar;32(1):50 – 56.

作者:Emilie J. B. Calvello

国际区域性疾病

156. Tetanus

1. Clinical Peal:

40 yo previously healthy male in China who presents with prolonged "seizure" after receiving a cut on his foot while fishing 5 days ago.

2. Dx: Tetanus.

3. Clinical features:

1) Incubation period 4 – 14 days

2) 3 clinical forms:

(1) Local spasm.

(2) Cephalic (rare)-cranial nerve involvement.

(3) Generalized (most common)-Descending spasm: facial sneer (risus sardonicus), "locked jaw" trismus, neck stiffness, laryngeal spasm, abdominal muscle spasm.

(4) Spasms continue to 3 – 4 weeks and can take months to fully recover.

4. Complications: apnea, rhabodymyolysis, fracture/dislocations.

5. Treatment: supportive, benzodiazepines, RSI, Tetanus IG (3000 – 5000 units IM), wound debridement.

Author: Emilie J. B. Calvello

156. 破伤风

1. 临床典型病例

40 岁健康中国男性，5 天前在钓鱼时脚上划了一个口子，现因长时间抽搐而来就诊。

2. 诊断：破伤风。

3. 临床表现

1) 潜伏期 4 ~ 14 天。

2) 3 种临床表现类型：

（1）局部痉挛。

（2）头部（罕见）：面部神经受侵袭。

（3）全身（最常见）下行性痉挛：面部抽搐性冷笑，牙关紧闭（锁颌），颈项强直，喉咽部痉挛，腹肌痉挛。

（4）痉挛性抽搐可持续 3 ~4 周，甚至几个月才能恢复。

4. 合并症：窒息、肌溶解综合症，骨折/关节脱位。

5. 治疗：支持疗法，苯二氮䓬类药物，气管插管，破伤风免疫球蛋白（3000 ~ 5000 单位肌注），伤口清创。

参考文献：

http：//www.cdc.gov/vaccines/pubs/pinkbook/tetanus.html

作者：**Emilie J. B. Calvello**

国际区域性疾病

371

157. Water Decontamination?

1. General Information:

Millions of people around the world (including our patients who travel and victims of disasters like Hurricane Sandy) are exposed to non-potable water.

2. How to treat contaminated water:

1) Filter cloudy water through a clean cloth or allow to settle prior to treatment.

2) The safest method is boiling water vigorously for 1 minute (or, at least 3 minutes at altitudes >6,000ft).

3) Chemical disinfection is not as effective, but, if boiling is unavailable use either:

(1) 2 drops of unscented bleach (5.52% Cl) per quart/liter of water. (Unknown strength? Add 10 drops per quart/liter.).

(2) Or 5 drops of tincture of 2% iodine per quart/liter.

4) If the water is cloudy or cold, double the chlorine or iodine.

3. Notes: Pregnant women or people with thyroid conditions should not use iodine.

4. UV decontamination can be accomplished by leaving clear bottles of water in direct sun for >6 hours or special equipment, but requires clear water.

5. Boiling, Chlorine/Iodine, and UV will kill viruses, bacteria, and Giardia

Only Boiling kills Cryptosporidium.

6. Bottom Line:

1) If bottled water is available, use it.

2) If not, boil your water.

3) In order to treat for a wide variety of pathogens, it is best to combine available methods.

Author: Andi Tenner

157. 污染水处理

1. 基本信息

全世界有数百万人饮用非饮用水，包括旅游者和像 Sandy 飓风这样的自然灾害的受害者。

2. 如何处理污染的水

1）处理前可用干净的衣服将浑浊的水过滤或放置沉淀。

2）最有效的方法是将水煮沸 1 分钟（如在海拔超过 1828 米的地方，至少需要 3 分钟）。

3）虽然化学处理不是同样有效，但在没有加热的条件下，可采用：

（1）每升水中加入 2 滴无味含 5.52% 氯或 10 滴不知氯浓度的漂白剂。

（2）或每升水中加入 5 滴含 2% 碘的碘酒。

4）如果水是浑浊或冷的，要放入双倍的氯或碘。

3. 注意：怀孕或有甲状腺问题的人不要用碘。

4. 利用紫外线消毒时，可将透明瓶子装的水放在阳光直晒处 6 小时以上，或用特殊的设备消毒，但水要清。

5. 煮沸、氯/碘或紫外线可杀死病毒、细菌和贾第鞭毛虫。

只有热沸腾才能杀死隐孢子虫。

6. 要点

1）争取饮用瓶装水。

2）如没有瓶装水，要将水煮沸

3）为达到更广泛的处理致病菌的效果，最好将上述方法联合使用。

参考文献：

United States Environmental Protection Agency. Water Health Series：Filtration Facts. 2005. http：//water. epa. gov/drink/info/upload/2005_11_17_faq_fs_healthseries_filtration. pdf. Accessed 11/27/12.

United States Environmental Protection Agenecy. Emergency Disinfection of Drinking Water. 2006. http：//water. epa. gov/drink/emerprep/emergencydisinfection. cfm. Accessed 11/27/12.

United States Center for Disease Control. Water Treatment Methods. 2011. http：//wwwnc. cdc. gov/travel/page/water-treatment. htm Accessed 11/27/12.

作者：**Andi Tenner**

国际区域性疾病

158. Soil based Helminth Infections)

1. More than 1.2 billion people are infected with at least one species.

2. Most helminth infections are contracted by ingesting the eggs, except strongyloides and hookworm whose larvae penetrate bare skin when it is contact with the soil.

3. The roundworm (Ascaris lumbricoides) life cycle involves migration through the lung tissue which can cause pneumonitis. Patients can present with interstitial infiltrates, wheeze, and blood tinged sputum. Ascaris then migrates to the intestines where it can cause partial small bowel obstruction. In pediatric patients, the appendix may be invaded causing gangrene with symptoms indistinguishable from appendicitis. In adults, the worms can invade the biliary tract and cause biliary disease or pancreatitis. Fever causes this helminth to migrate and it can emerge from the nasopharynx or the anus.

4. Whipworms (Trichuris trichiura) present as colitis or symptoms similar to inflammatory bowel disease. Chronic illness can involve anemia and clubbing. In severe cases, trichuris can cause dysentery and rectal prolapse.

5. Hookworms (Necator americanus or Ancylostoma duodenale) also have a pulmonary phase, but with milder symptoms than Ascaris. Eventually hookworms cause iron deficiency anemia and malnutrition. They can be a primary cause of anemia in pregnancy in endemic areas.

6. Threadworm (Strongyloides stercoralis) can cause a wide spectrum of disease presentations. The infection can start with a rash, larva currens. The infection may be subclinical or may invade the lung, intestinal wall, or the nervous system. Eventually hyperinfection may develop which is a very large increase in worm burden and then the infection becomes disseminated.

7. Toxocara canis or toxocara cati have affected approximately 14% of the US population. These helminthes reproduce in dogs or cats, and human infection is not part of the normal life cycle. Most infections are subclinical but it can produce a mild pneumonitis that is very similar to asthma. There can be pain and inflammation as the helminthes travel through organs such as the liver or lung and is called visceral larva migrans. The helminth may also move through the eye and optic never causing an ocular form of the disease, ocular larva migrans.

8. Pinworms (Enterobius vermicularis) are the cause of most common helminth infection in US and can present with anal pruritus leading to trouble sleeping. When an infection is identified, everyone in the household should be treated, regardless of symptoms.

Author: Jenny Reifel Saltzberg

国
际
区
域
性
疾
病

158. 土源性蠕虫感染

1. 超过 12 亿的人有至少一次的蠕虫感染史。

2. 最常见的蠕虫感染途径是摄入虫卵，但线虫和钩虫感染是由人类皮肤与含有其幼虫的土壤接触所致。

3. 蛔虫（Ascaris lumbricoides）生命周期包括：迁移到肺部，造成肺炎，患者可有肺侵润、哮喘和痰中带血的表现。然后，蛔虫会迁徙到肠道，造成部分小肠梗阻。在儿童患者中，蛔虫可侵入阑尾造成与阑尾炎难以分辨的坏疽。对成人而言，蛔虫可侵入胆道导致胆道系统疾病和胰腺炎。发热可促进蠕虫的迁徙，使其由鼻咽或肛门排出。

4. 鞭虫（Trichuris trichiura）感染者可出现结肠炎或与炎性肠病类似的症状。慢性感染者可出现贫血和杵状指。重症患者可出现痢疾和直肠脱垂。

5. 钩虫（Necator americanus or Ancylostoma duodenale）也可影响肺部，只是症状要比蛔虫轻。最终会导致缺铁性贫血和营养不良。它们可能是流行区妊娠期贫血的主要原因。

6. 线虫（Strongyloides stercoralis）的临床表现相当广泛，早期可有皮疹、幼虫移行症。感染可以是亚临床性，也可侵润到肺、肠壁或神经系统。最终会出现高度传染，蠕虫的大量快速增殖导致感染的扩散。

7. 犬弓首线虫或猫弓首线虫已感染了大约 14% 的美国人口。这些蠕虫在狗或猫体内繁殖，人类感染不是其正常生命周期的一部分。许多感染都是亚临床的，但可出现类似哮喘的轻型肺炎。当蠕虫移动于各器官时（如肝脏或肺）可产生疼痛和炎症，这一过程叫内脏蠕虫蚴移行症。蠕虫也可能迁移到眼睛和视神经，导致眼部疾病，即眼部蠕虫蚴移行症。

8. 蛲虫（Enterobius vermicularis）是美国最常见的蠕虫感染，表现为影响睡眠的肛门瘙痒。如确定感染，不论有无症状，家里的每个人都要接受治疗。

参考文献：

J Bethony, S Brooker, M Albonico, S M Geiger, A Loukas, D Diemert, P J Hotez. Soil-transmitted helminth infections: ascariasis, trichuriasis, and hookworm. Lancet: 2006; 367: 1521 – 1532.

S Knopp, P Steinmann, J Keiser, J Utzinger. Nematode Infections: Soil-Transmitted Helminths and Trichinella Infect Dis Clin N Am: 2012; 26: 341 – 358.

作者: **Jenny Reifel Saltzberg**

国
际
区
域
性
疾
病

159. Glucose 6 Phosphate Dehydrogenase deficiency

1. The most common disease producing enzymopathy in humans.

2. Affects 400 million people worldwide.

3. Highest prevalence is among persons of African, Asian, and Mediterranean descent.

4. Patients can be asymptomatic but may present with symptoms of acute hemolytic anemia, which may be precipitated by certain medications (Oxidative medications) or foods (some types of beans).

5. Avoid oxidative drugs (consult your PharmD when your patient has G6PDd).

6. Diagnosis: Measure the actual enzyme activity of G6PD rather than the amount of the enzyme. A more practical test is the presence of Indirect hyperbilirubinemia, but it is non specific.

7. Treatment consists of oxygen and bed rest in minor cases. However, severe cases may require PRBC transfusion.

Author: Walid Hammad

159. 葡萄糖－6 磷酸脱氢酶缺乏

1. 葡萄糖－6 磷酸脱氢酶缺乏(G6PDd)是人类最常见的酶缺乏病。

2. 全世界有 4 亿人受影响。

3. 最高发患者群是非洲人、亚洲人和地中海后裔。

4. 患者可能没有症状，或可有急性溶血性贫血的表现。症状可由一些药物(氧化性药物)或食物(某些豆类)引起。

5. 避免氧化性药物(遇到有 G6PDd 的患者要与药剂师咨询)。

6. 诊断：测定 G6PD 酶活性而不是酶的量。另外一个较实用的实验是间接高胆红素血症，但它不特异。

7. 如病情轻，治疗上可只给氧和卧床休息，但严重者可能需要输血。

参考文献：

Beutler E. Glucose－6－phosphate dehydrogenase deficiency：a historical perspective. Blood. Jan 1 2008；111(1)：16－24.

Nkhoma ET, Poole C, Vannappagari V, et al. The global prevalence of glucose-6-phosphate dehydrogenase deficiency：a systematic review and meta-analysis. Blood Cells Mol Dis. May－Jun 2009；42(3)：267－278.

作者：**Walid Hammad**

国际区域性疾病

160. Japanese Encephalitis

1. General Information:

1) caused by Japanese encephalitis virus (JEV), closely related to West Nile virus.

2) transmission is through infected mosquito.

3) most common cause of vaccine-preventable cause of encephalitis in Asia.

4) Incubation period is 5 – 15 days.

5) <1% develop clinical, disease, most asymptomatic.

6) Acute encephalitis most common presentation.

7) Sx: altered mental status, focal neuro deficits, movement disorder, seizure, fever, headache, vomiting.

8) Classic presentation: Parkinsonian syndrome with mask-like facies, tremor, cogwheel rigidity, and choreoathetoid movements.

9) case-fatality is 20% – 30%.

2. Area of the world affected:

Primarily in Asia-China, Japan, Korea, India, Southeast Asia.

3. Relevance to the US physician:

1) General

Should be considered in patients concerned for neurological infection with recent travel to endemic country.

2) Lab: JEV-specific IgM in serum (after 7 days of sx onset) or CSF (after 4 days of sx onset).

Viral culture and other viral RNA amplifications tests are not sensitive.

3) Treatment is supportive.

4) In survivors, 30 – 50% have significant neurological, cognitive, psychological sequelae.

5) Vaccine.

One vaccine (Ixiaro) is available in the US.

(1) 2 doses, 28 days apart (96% develop immunity).

(2) No information on duration of protection.

(3) Recommended for travelers ≥1 month in endemic areas during JEV season.

4. Bottom Line：

Very rare but deadly disease with high mortality and post-infection sequelae. Think about it in travelers to Asia during summer/fall seasons who have not been immunized.

Author：Andrea Tenner, Veronic Pei

160. 日本脑炎

1. 基本概况

1）由与西尼罗河病毒亲缘密切的日本脑炎病毒感染引起。

2）由感染的蚊子传播。

3）是亚洲最常见的能够由疫苗预防的脑炎。

4）潜伏期为 5～15 天。

5）多数患者无症状，只有低于 1% 的患者有临床表现。

6）急性脑炎是最常见的表现。

7）症状：神志改变、局部神经功能丧失、运动失调、癫痫、发热、头痛、呕吐。

8）典型表现：帕金森综合征的表现，假面状容貌、颤抖、齿轮样强直和舞蹈手足徐动症。

9）死亡率为 20%～30%。

2. 世界流行地区

主要在亚洲，包括中国、日本、韩国、印度、东南亚。

3. 美国医生要注意什么

1）常识

对怀疑有神经系统感染并在最近到过流行区旅游的患者要考虑此病。

2）实验室检查：日本脑炎病毒（JEV）：血清特异性 IgM（起病后 7 天内）或 CSF IgM（起病后 4 天内）。

病毒培养和其他病毒 RNA 放大实验并不敏感。

3）治疗：主要是支持治疗。

4）在幸存者中，30%～50% 会有明显的神经、认知和心理方面的后遗症。

5）疫苗

美国有一种疫苗（乙型脑炎灭活疫苗）：

（1）要接种两次，相隔 28 天（96% 产生免疫力）；

（2）没有有关保护期的资料；

（3）建议高发季节到流行区旅游超过 1 个月以上的旅游者接种。

4. 要点

日本脑炎是一种罕见但具有高死亡率和感染后后遗症的恶性疾病。对在夏秋季到亚洲且没有免疫力的旅游者要考虑此病。

参考文献：

http：//wwwnc. cdc. gov/travel/yellowbook/2012/chapter-3-infectious-diseases-related-to-travel/japanese-encephalitis. htm#2473

作者：**Andrea Tenner，Veronic Pei**

国
际
区
域
性
疾
病

161. New SARS-Like Virus

1. General Information:

14 cases of lower respiratory infection caused by a new coronavirus (not the original SARS virus, but with a similar picture) occurred in 2013. Mortality rate of this virus is >50%.

2. Area of the world affected:

1) Arabian Peninsula.

2) United Kingdom.

3. Relevance to us:

1) Suspect this with a lower respiratory tract infection not responding to therapy and a travel history.

2) Person to person transmission possible.

3) Can have coinfection with influenza.

4) PCR testing can be done at the CDC in suspected cases.

4. Bottom Line:

1) Consider this infection in patients with a lower respiratory tract infection who have traveled to or had contact with someone who traveled to the above regions in the past 10 days.

2) ASK ABOUT RECENT TRAVELS IN PATIENTS PRESENTING WITH SYMPTOMS OF SEVERE LOWER RESPIRATORY TRACT INFECTION!

Author: Andrea Tenner and Veronica Pei

161. 新型类 SARS 病毒

1. 基本信息

2013 年一共出现了 14 例由一种新型的冠状病毒(与 SARS 病毒不一样,但相似)导致的下呼吸道感染病例。这种病毒感染的死亡率超过 50%。

2. 国际影响区域

1)阿拉伯半岛;

2)英国。

3. 与我们的关系

1)对常规治疗无反应并有旅游经历的下呼吸道感染患者,要怀疑此病毒感染。

2)可以经过人与人传播。

3)可以与流感病毒同时感染。

4)对可疑患者,疾病控制中心可做 PCR 试验。

4. 要点

1)对在 10 天内到过上述地区或与到过上述地区的人有过接触,并患有下呼吸道感染的患者要考虑到这一感染的可能。

2)对严重下呼吸道感染的患者,一定要问近期旅游史!

参考文献:

http://www.cdc.gov/mmwr/preview/mmwrhtml/mm6210a4.htm?s_cid=mm6210a4_w

作者: Andrea Tenner and Veronica Pei

国际区域性疾病

385

162. Acute and Potentially Life-Threatening Tropical Diseases in Western Travelers-A GeoSentinel Multicenter Study, 1996—2011

1. Background Information:

1) Each year, an estimated 50 million travelers from Western countries visit tropical regions all over the world.

2) Given the potentially serious consequences for the patients and, their close contacts and healthcare workers it is important that life threatening tropical diseases are swiftly diagnosed.

2. Pertinent Study Design and Conclusions:

1) Descriptive analysis of acute and potentially life threatening tropical diseases among 82, 825 ill western travelers reported to GeoSentinel from June of 1996 to August of 2011.

2) Of these travelers, 3, 655 (4.4%) patients had an acute and potentially life threatening disease.

3) The four most common conditions being falciparum malaria (76.9%), typhoid fever (11.7%), paratyphoid fever (6.4%), and leptospirosis (2.4%).

3. Bottom Line:

Western physicians seeing febrile and recently returned travelers from the tropics need to consider a wide profile of potentially life threatening tropical illnesses, with a specific focus on the most likely diseases described in this case series.

Author: Walid Hammad

美国急诊临床必知200招

162. 1996—2011 年热带疾病对西方游客的威胁 ——来自 GeoSentinel 中心的研究

1. 背景资料

1)每年估计有 5 000 万来自西方国家的游客游览世界各地的热带地区。

2)致命的热带病可给患者、密切接触者和医务工作者带来潜在的严重后果，因此快速诊断是非常重要的。

2. 相关的研究设计和结论

1)这是一个对从 1996 年 6 月至 2011 年 8 月通过 GeoSentinel 登记的 82 825 名西方旅游者中患有急性和潜在致命的热带疾病的描述性分析报告。

2)在这些旅客中，有 3 655 例(4.4%)患有急性和潜在致命的疾病。

3)四种最常见的疾病是恶性疟疾(76.9%)，伤寒(11.7%)，副伤寒(6.4%)和钩端螺旋体病(2.4%)。

3. 要点

西方医生在接诊最近从热带地区返回的发热旅客时需考虑许多潜在致命的热带疾病，尤其要注意上面谈到的最有可能的疾病。

参考文献：

Jensenius M, Han PV, Schlagenhauf P, Schwartz E, Parola P, Castelli F, von Sonnenburg F, Loutan L, Leder K, Freedman DO; GeoSentinel Surveillance Network. Acute and potentially life-threatening tropical diseases in western travelers—a GeoSentinel multicenter study, 1996 – 2011. Am J Trop Med Hyg. 2013 Feb; 88(2): 397 – 404

国际区域性疾病

163. Global Health Policy—The Big Picture

1. General Information

1) The global health world is faced with an unprecedented challenge of a trio of threats:

Infections, undernutrition, reproductive health issues.

2) Rising global burden of non-communicable diseases and risk factors.

3) Challenges arising from globalization (climate change and trade politics).

2. Definitions of global health are variable and can emphasize anything from types of health problems, populations of interest, geographic area or a specific mission. This makes governance and analysis difficult.

3. During the past decade there has been an explosion of more than 175 initiatives, funds, agencies, and donors. Health is increasingly influenced by decisions made in other global policymaking areas.

4. The major governance challenges for global health are:

1) Defining national sovereignty in the context of deepening health interdependence.

2) Maximizing cross-sector interdependence.

3) Developing clear mechanisms of accountability for non-state actors.

5. Relevance to the US physician

The Global Health System and its governance affects our ability to work effectively within the US and how we structure efforts to expand the reach of timely, effective emergency care worldwide.

6. Bottom Line

The Global Health System has become more complex. Any development of Emergency Care Systems must take into account the complexity of actors in the field of global health.

Author: Andrea Tenner

163. 全球健康政策——宏观规划

1. 一般资料

1）全球健康领域正在面临前所未有的三个威胁：

感染、营养不良、生殖健康问题。

2）快速增长的非传染性疾病及其危险因素。

3）全球化的挑战（气候的变化和贸易政策）。

2. 全球健康的定义差异很大，但可强调包括健康问题的类型、人群利益、地理位置或一个特别论题的任何内容。这就导致了管理和分析上的困难。

3. 在过去十年中爆炸性的涌出了超过 175 个倡议、基金、机构和捐助者。全球其他领域所作出的决定对健康的影响越来越明显。

4. 全球健康管理面临的主要挑战

1）在深化医药卫生相互依存的背景下定义国家主权。

2）跨部门的相互依存最大化。

3）为非国家行为制定明确的责任制。

5. 与美国医生的关系

全球健康体系和治理影响医生们的工作效率，我们应考虑如何规划和努力扩展及时有效的全球紧急医疗体系。

6. 要点

全球健康体系已经变得更加复杂。在筹建任何紧急救护系统时必须要考虑到全球健康领域所有参与者的复杂性。

参考文献：

An interactive graphic can be found at：http：//www. nejm. org/doi/full/10. 1056/NEJM-ra1109339？query = featured_home

Frenk，J. and Moon，S. Governance Challenges in Global Health. NEJM 2013；368：936 – 942.

作者：**Andrea Tenner**

国际区域性疾病

药物中毒
Toxicology

164. Highlights from the new
Salicylate Toxicity Management Guideline 2013

In June 2013 the American College of Medical Toxicology (ACMT) released a Guidance Document on the Management Priorities in Salicylate Toxicity. Here are some key highlights:

1)Continuous IV infusion of sodium bicarbonate is indicated even in the presence of mild alkalemia from the early respiratory alkalosis.

2)Euvolemia is important.

3)If intubation is required, administration of sodium bicarbonate by IV bolus at the time of intubation in a sufficient quantity to maintain a blood pH of 7.45 - 7.5 over the next 30 minutes is a reasonable management option during this critical juncture.

4)Once airway control has been established, it is imperative that the increased minute ventilation and low PCO2 usually seen with salicylate intoxication are maintained.

5)A salicylate concentration approaching 100 mg/dL warrants consideration of hemodialysis in the acute toxicity setting (40 mg/dL for chronic toxicity). Consult nephrology well before these threshold levels.

Author: Bryan Hayes

164. 2013 年水杨酸中毒处理指南

美国医学毒理学学院(ACMT)在 2013 年 6 月发布了如何处理水杨酸中毒的指南文件。要点如下：

1)即使在早期存在由呼吸性碱中毒造成的碱中毒情况下，也要持续静脉滴注碳酸氢钠。

2)体液平衡很重要。

3)如果需要插管，在插管时要静脉推注足够量的碳酸氢钠使其能够在接下来的 30 分钟内保持血液 pH 在 7.45 ~ 7.5。这是在这种关键情况下的合理处理方案。

4)一旦气道控制已经建立，要注意维持水杨酸中毒时常见的高每分钟通气量和低二氧化碳分压。

5)在急性中毒时，如水杨酸浓度接近 7.25 mmol/L，要积极考虑血液透析(慢性中毒为 2.90 mmol/L)，要在药物血液浓度水平达到这些阈值前请肾脏科会诊。

参考文献：

Guidance Document：Management Priorities in Salicylate Toxicity

http：//www. acmt. net/cgi/page. cgi/zine_service. html？aid = 4210&zine = show

作者：Bryan Hayes

药
物
中
毒

165. Acetaminophen Toxicity-When Should I Consider Liver Transplant?

1. If you are working in a community hospital and have an acetaminophen overdose, one of the criteria to transfer the patient to a tertiary care center is presence of the King's College Criteria.

2. Each one is assigned points and can be prognostic for severe toxicity and need for transplant. The lactate and phosphorus are new ones and have modified the criteria. Phosphorus is utilized to create glycogen. If the liver is injured and trying to heal, your phosphorus will be low (good). If the liver is injured and unable to repair itself the phosphorus will be high (bad). This single test has an excellent prognostic ability.

1) Lactate > 3.5 mg/dL (0.39 mmol/L) 4 hrs after early fluid resuscitation?

2) pH < 7.30 or lactate > 3 mg/dL (0.33 mmol/L) after full fluid resuscitation at 12 hours.

3) INR > 6.5 (PTT $> 100s$).

4) Creatinine > 3.4 mg/dL (300 μmol/L).

5) Phosphorus > 3.75 mg/dL (1.2 mmol/L) at 48 hours.

Author: Fermin Barrueto

165. 对乙酰氨基酚中毒是否需要考虑肝移植？

1. 如果你在社区医院工作，接诊一位对乙酰氨基酚用药过量的患者，将患者转移至三级医疗中心的标准之一是 King College 标准。

2. 每一个指标有一个分数标准，可以用来判断中毒的严重程度和是否需要移植。乳酸和磷是修改后的新指标，糖原的形成需要磷。肝脏受伤时，如有愈合倾向，血磷会降低（好现象）；如果肝脏受伤而无法自我修复时，血磷会升高（坏现象）。这是一个很好的预后预测的单一指标。

1）早期液体复苏 4 小时后，乳酸 >0.39 mmol/L；

2）在液体复苏 12 小时后，pH <7.30 或乳酸 >3.4 mg/dL（0.33 mmol/L）

3）INR >6.5 s；

4）肌酐 73.4 mg/dL（30 μmol/L）；

5）48 小时后磷 >3.5 mg/dL（1.2 mmol/L）。

参考文献：

http：//www. mdcalc. com/kings-college-criteria-for-acetaminophen-toxicity/

作者：**Fermin Barrueto**

药
物
中
毒

166. Effect of N-Acetylcysteine on Prothrombin Time and Coagulation Factors

1. In the treatment of acetaminophen poisoning with N-acetylcysteine (NAC), the PT/INR can be slightly elevated even in the absence of hepatotoxicity. Considering Prothombin Time (PT) is one of the criteria used to assess severity of liver damage in this setting, it is important to know how much the PT/INR can be affected by NAC and if it has an actual effect on coagulation factor levels.

1) N-acetylcysteine has been shown to slightly increase the PT by up to 3.5 seconds in healthy volunteers.

2) A more recent study by the same authors demonstrated a reduction in vitamin K-dependent clotting factor activity (II, VI, IX, and X) after NAC administration in healthy volunteers.

2. Clinical Practice Pearls

1) The elevation in PT/INR after NAC administration is real, not simply laboratory interference.

2) However, the PT/INR elevation and decrease in coagulation factors is modest and not likely clinical significant.

3) Many poison center guidelines allow for an INR up to 2 to be considered 'normal' to account for this phenomenon in this setting.

Author: Bryan Hayes

166. N-乙酰半胱氨酸对凝血酶原时间和凝血因子的影响

1. 用 N-乙酰半胱氨酸（NAC）治疗对乙酰氨基酚中毒时，即使没有肝毒性，PT/INR也可以略有升高。由于凝血酶原时间（PT）是用来评估在此情况下肝损害严重程度的标准之一，因此知道 NAC 可使 PT/INR 增高多少和它对凝血因子水平的影响是重要的。

1）研究显示，在健康志愿者中，N-乙酰半胱氨酸可使 PT 增高至 3.5 秒。

2）相同作者最近的研究表明，健康志愿者在用 NAC 后维生素 K 依赖性凝血因子的活性（Ⅱ，Ⅵ，Ⅸ，Ⅹ）降低。

2. 临床实践要点

1）用 NAC 后 PT/INR 升高是客观存在的，并非简单的由实验室误差造成；

2）然而，PT/INR 增高和凝血因子减少是轻微的，很可能没有什么临床意义；

3）在这种情形下，许多中心的指南将 INR 为 2 视为"正常"。

参考文献：

Pizon AF, et al. The in vitro effect of n-acetylcysteine on prothrombin time in plasma samples from healthy subjects. Acad Emerg Med 2011; 18: 351 – 354.

Jang DH, et al. In vitro study of n-acetylcysteine on coagulation factors in plasma samples from healthy subjects. J Med Tox 2013; 9: 49 – 53.

作者：**Bryan Hayes**

167. Gastric Lavage: Position Paper Update

In 2013, the American Academy of Clinical Toxicology and European Association of Poisons Centres and Clinical Toxicologists published a second update to their position statement on gastric lavage for GI decontamination (original 1997, 1st update 2004). Here are the highlights:

1) Gastric lavage should not be performed routinely, if at all, for the treatment of poisoned patients.

2) Further, the evidence supporting gastric lavage as a beneficial treatment even in special situations is weak.

3) In the rare instances in which gastric lavage is indicated, it should only be performed by individuals with proper training and expertise.

Gastric lavage generally causes more harm than good. It should not be thought of as a viable GI decontamination method.

Author: Bryan Hayes

167. 洗胃

2013 年 2 月美国临床毒理学学会和欧洲毒物中心和临床毒理学协会联合发表了第二个洗胃在清除胃肠毒物时应用价值的声明(原始版在 1997 年, 2004 年第一次更新)。要点如下:

1)洗胃不应该作为治疗中毒患者的常规手段。

2)另外, 在某些特殊情况下支持洗胃有效应用的证据也是缺乏的。

3)即使在罕见情况下确实需要洗胃, 也要由经过培训并有经验的人员来操作。

通常来讲, 洗胃的害处多于益处, 它不应该被认为是一种有效的清除胃肠毒物的方法。

参考文献:

Benson BE, et al. Position paper update: gastric lavage for gastrointestinal decontamination. Clin Toxicol 2013 Feb 18. [Epub ahead of print]

作者: **Bryan Hayes**

药
物
中
毒

168. Digoxin Toxicity With Normal Digoxin Levels

1. Digoxin toxicity can occur in patients with normal digoxin levels. In patients taking digoxin in recommended doses, digoxin toxicity can occur in the setting of hypokalemia or hypomagnesemia, even though the serum digoxin level is within normal limits.

2. Digoxin directly inhibits the sodium-potassium ATPase pump in the membrane of the cardiac myocyte, causing an increase in intracellular sodium and calcium which increases myocardial contractility.

3. Hypokalemia increases digoxin cardiac sensitivity because potassium and digoxin compete for the same ATPase-binding site. Magnesium is a cofactor of the sodium-potassium ATPase pump. Hypomagnesemia increases myocardial digoxin uptake, further inhibiting sodium-potassium ATPase pump activity.

4. It is known that long-term digoxin users often have hypokalemia or hypomagnesemia, presumably due to diuretic usage in patients with congestive heart failure.

5. In a suggestive clinical setting, do not exclude the possibility of digoxin toxicity simply because the digoxin level is in the therapeutic range, and be sure to check serum potassium and magnesium levels.

Author: Feng Xiao

168. 正常浓度下的地高辛中毒

1.服用推荐剂量的地高辛患者，即使血清地高辛浓度在正常范围内，也可发生地高辛中毒。地高辛中毒还可在低钾血症或低镁血症的情况下发生。

2.地高辛直接抑制心肌细胞膜的钠－钾 ATP 酶，导致细胞内的钠和钙的增加，进而增加心肌收缩力。

3.由于钾和地高辛竞争同样的 ATP 酶结合位点，低钾血症会增加心脏对地高辛的敏感度。镁是钠－钾 ATP 酶的辅助因子，因此低镁血症会增加心肌对地高辛的吸收，进一步抑制钠－钾 ATP 酶的活性。

4.众所周知，长期使用地高辛的患者往往有低钾或低镁血症，可能是因为充血性心力衰竭患者多使用利尿药。

5.在临床怀疑地高辛中毒情况下，不要因为地高辛浓度在正常范围内就排除这种可能性，一定要检查血清中钾和镁的水平。

参考文献：

Raja Rao MP, et al. J Emerg Med 2013；epub，May 20，2013.

Dec GW. Med Clin North Am 2003；87；317－337.

Chan KE, et al. J Am SocNephrol 2010；21：1550－1559.

作者：**Feng Xiao**

药
物
中
毒

169. Cocaine-Induced Abdominal Pain

1. The well-known effects ofcocaine toxicity include seizures, cardiac ischemia, and rhabdomyolysis. Abdominal pain, however, is a lesser known side-effect and may occur secondaryto ischemia, infarction or perforation of the gastrointestinal tract; such-cases tend to occur in younger people without known risk factors for ischemia.

2. Ischemia may occur from thedirect vasoconstrictive effects of cocaine, but may also occur from itspro-thrombotic effects on the mesenteric vessels; although any segment of theGI tract may be involved, the small bowel is most often affected.

3. Symptoms may vary from mildabdominal pain to bloody diarrhea. Physical exam may reveal peritoneal signs ifperforation occurs.

4. CT scan of the abdomen mayreveal the diagnosis although angiography may required for diagnosis or toguide revascularization.

5. Management may vary fromconservative (i. e. , bowel rest and antibiotics) to surgical exploration andbowel resection in selected cases.

Author: **HaneyMallemat**

169. 可卡因引起的腹痛

1.可卡因的毒性效应是众所周知的,包括癫痫发作、心肌缺血和横纹肌溶解。而腹痛是一个不太为人知的不良反应,其出现可能是由于继发的胃肠道缺血、梗塞或穿孔,这通常发生在没有缺血危险因素的年轻人中。

2.缺血可能与可卡因的直接收缩血管作用有关,但也可由肠系膜血管促血栓形成效应引起,虽然可能发生在胃肠道的任何部分,但小肠是最常见的受累部位。

3.症状可从轻微腹痛到血性腹泻,如果发生穿孔,可有腹膜炎体征。

4.腹部 CT 扫描可确诊,但偶尔需要血管造影来确诊或指导血管重建。

5.可以保守治疗(即肠道休息和抗生素),某些病例可能要手术探查和肠道切除。

参考文献:

Zimmerman, J. Cocaine intoxication[J]. Crit Care Clinics, 2012 Oct; 28(4): 517 – 526.

作者: HaneyMallemat

药物中毒

170. Lipid Emulsion Therapy: Current Status

1. Emergency Physicians should be aware that lipid emulsion therapy, which was once considered experimental, is now a mainstream therapy being used with increasing frequency.

2. A recent survey of US Poison Control Centers revealed that most have a protocol for LE therapy (1). In a scenario with "cardiac arrest" due to a single agent, PCC directors stated that their center would "always" or "often" recommend LE therapy after overdose of bupivacaine (96%), verapamil (80%), amitriptyline (69%), or an unknown agent (27%).

3. In a scenario with "shock", directors stated that their PCC would "always" or "often" recommend LE therapy after overdose of bupivacaine (89%), verapamil (62%), amitriptyline (56%), or an unknown agent (18%).

4. Most directors feel that LE is safe but are more likely to recommend LE therapy in patients with cardiac arrest than in patients with severe hemodynamic compromise.

5. The majority of PCCs recommend an initial bolus of 20% lipid emulsion at a dose of 1.5 mL/kg. The bolus is followed by an infusion at a rate of 0.25 ml/kg/min.

6. Clinicians should be aware that LE therapy interferes with some laboratory measurements (2). Serum glucose concentrations when determined by colorimetric testing and serum magnesium and albumin concentrations become inaccurate following the administration of LE, while creatinine, lipase, ALT, CK and bilirubin become unmeasurable.

Author: EMedHome. com

美
国
急
诊
临
床
必
知
200
招

170. 脂肪乳剂治疗现状

1. 急诊医师应该知道，曾经被认为是实验性的脂肪乳剂（LE）治疗，现在已是一种使用频率越来越高的主要治疗方法。

2. 美国毒物控制中心（PCC）最近的一项调查表明，大多数中心都有使用 LE 治疗指南。在单个药物导致"心脏骤停"的情况下，PCC 主任们表示，他们的中心"总是"或"经常"推荐用 LE 治疗因过量服用布比卡因（96%）、维拉帕米（80%）、阿米替林（69%）或单一未知药物（27%）过量带来的问题。

3. 在"休克"的情况下，主任们表示他们的 PCC"总是"或"经常"推荐用 LE 治疗因过量服用布比卡因（89%）、维拉帕米（62%）、阿米替林（56%）或单一未知药物（18%）过量带来的问题。

4. 大多数主任认为 LE 是安全的，与严重的血流动力学紊乱相比患者，他们更倾向于在心脏骤停患者中应用 LE。

5. 大多数 PCC 建议初始注射剂量为 1.5 mL/kg 20% 的脂肪乳剂。然后以 0.25 mL/(kg·min) 的速度静脉注射。

临床医生应该了解 LE 疗法会干扰某些实验室检查。应用 LE 后，比色法检测的血清葡萄糖浓度和血清镁和白蛋白浓度会不准确，而脂肪酶、肌酐、ALT、CK 和胆红素会变得测不到。

参考文献：

Christian MR, et al. J Med Toxicol 2013 May 10. ［Epub ahead of print］

Grunbaum AM, et al. Clin Toxicol (Phila) 2012；50：812 – 817.

作者：EMedHome.com

药物中毒

171. Lipid Emulsion
Therapy-Increasing Evidence

1. Utilizing 20% lipid emulsion at a dose of 1.5 mL/kg (100 mL Bolus) IV with repeat in 15 minutes in no response is being recommended in patients hemodynamic instabiity due to poisoning.

2. Probably more effective in lipophilic drugs is a current theory for the mechanism of action-the "lipid sink". The idea is that the lipids envelope the drug pulling it off its receptors or sequestering it in the intravascular space. A recent paper has added another mechanism-direct inotropic and lusiptropic effects.

3. Also, if you think the therapy is experimental, think again. Another recent paper surveyed Poison Control Centers and found 30/45 Poison Centers in the US have a defined protocol for utilization of lipid emulsion therapy. The PCCs are recommending it more.

4. What was once considered just a purely experimental therapy only used at the very end of code is becoming more mainstream. Comfort with its safety profile and efficacy continues to mount.

Author: Fermin Barrueto

美
国
急
诊
临
床
必
知
200
招

171. 脂肪乳剂治疗——新的证据

1. 在抢救血流动力学不稳定的中毒患者时，可用 1.5 mL/kg（100 毫静推）20% 的脂肪乳剂，如没有反应可在 15 分钟内按同样剂量重复一次。

2. 对亲脂性药物更有效可能是因为其作用机理 - "脂肪沉淀"，这一机理是脂质将药物包裹使其与药物受体分离或沉淀在血管内。最近的一篇论文谈到了另外一种机制——直接的肌力增强效果。

3. 另外，如果你认为这种治疗还是处于实验阶段，多思考一下。最近的一篇论文对美国毒物控制中心进行了调查，发现美国 30/45 毒物中心有明确的脂肪乳剂，美国毒物控制中心越来越多的推荐它。

4. 这种曾经被认为只是用于抢救末期患者的实验性治疗将成为主要的抢救手段。对其安全性和效果的认知将会继续增加。

参考文献：

Fettiplace MR，Ripper R，Lis K，Lin B，Lang J，Zider B，Wang J，Rubinstein I，Weinberg G. Rapid Cardiotonic Effects of Lipid Emulsion Infusion. Crit Care Med. 2013 Mar 25.［Epub ahead of print］

Christian MR，Pallasch EM，Wahl M，Mycyk MB. Lipid Rescue 911：Are Poison Centers Recommending Intravenous Fat Emulsion Therapy for Severe Poisoning? J Med Toxicol. 2013 May 10. ［Epub ahead of print］

作者：Fermin Barrueto

药物中毒

172. Intravenous Lipid Emulsion for Cardiac Toxicity

1. Common life-threatening cardiovascular effects of cocaine intoxication include tachydysrhythmias, ventricular fibrillation, myocardial ischemia, and infarction.

2. Emergency management of acute cocaine intoxication relies mainly on supportive and symptomatic treatment, w/liberal use of gamma-aminobutyric acid receptor agonists such as benzodiazepines.

3. Intravenous lipid emulsion (ILE) therapy has been used successfully to treat cardiac toxicity associated with a variety of lipid-soluble drugs, such as local anesthetics, calcium/beta-blockers, tricyclic anti-depressants, and cocaine.

4. The current hypothesis, called the "lipid sink" hypothesis, suggest that ILE infusion creates an expanded lipid phase in the plasma that absorbs the circulating lipophilic toxin and decreases the amount of free unbound toxin available to bind to the myocardium.

5. When life-threatening cardiac arrhythmias (e. g. wide-complex tachycardia/prolonged QT) are not amenable to standard therapy (e. g. sodium bicarbonate/magnesium) consider ILE as a potential option to the current algorithm.

Author: Semhar Tewelde

172. 静脉注射脂肪乳对抗可卡因的心脏毒性

1. 可卡因常见的致死性的心血管效应包括快速性心率紊乱、心室颤动、心肌缺血和心肌梗死。

2. 急性可卡因中毒的急诊抢救主要依赖于支持疗法和改善症状及应用 γ－氨基丁酸受体兴奋剂，如苯二氮䓬类药物。

3. 静脉注射脂肪乳已被成功地用来治疗许多脂溶性药物所致的心脏毒性，如局部麻醉药、钙/β 受体阻滞药、三环类抗抑郁药和可卡因。

4. 目前所谓的"脂肪沉淀"假设理论，提出静脉注射脂肪乳将增加可吸收循环中亲脂性毒素的血浆脂质含量，进而减少可能与心肌结合的游离毒素量。

5. 对危及生命的心律失常（如宽 QRS 室速/QT 延长）在常规治疗（碳酸氢钠和镁）无效时，可考虑将静脉注射脂肪乳作为一种有潜力的治疗方案。

参考文献：

Arora N，Berk W，et al. Usefulness of Intravenous Lipid Emulsion for Cardiac Toxicity from Cocaine Overdose. The American Journal of Cardiology. Volume 111，Issue 3. Feb 2013.

作者：**Semhar Tewelde**

药物中毒

173. Antidote Safety in Pregnancy

1. Most antidotes have not been adequately studied in pregancy and hold a Pregnancy Risk Category 'C' by the FDA. However, there are a few antidotes that hold a category 'D' or 'X' rating (contraindicated).

2. Ethanol (toxic alcohols)-Category C

1) Reproduction studies have not been conducted with alcohol injection. Ethanol crosses the placenta, enters the fetal circulation, and has teratogenic effects in humans. When used as an antidote during the second or third trimester, Fetal Alcohol Syndrome AS is not likely to occur due to the short treatment period; use during the first trimester is controversial.

2) Alternative (preferred) antidote: fomepizole.

3. Methylene blue (methemoglobinemia)-Category X

Use during amniocentesis has shown evidence of fetal abnormalities, but it has been used orally without similar adverse events. IV may be ok.

4. Lorazepam and diazepam (seizures, nerve agents)-Category D

Teratogenic effects have been observed in some animal studies and in humans. Lorazepam/diazepam and their metabolite cross the human placenta.

5. Potassium iodide (radioactive iodine)-Category D

Iodide crosses the placenta (may cause hypothyroidism and goiter in fetus/newborn). Use for protection against thyroid cancer secondary to radioactive iodine exposure is considered acceptable based upon risk: benefit, keeping in mind the dose and duration.

6. Amyl nitrite (cyanide)- Category C (manufacturer contraindicates)

1) Animal reproduction studies have not been conducted. Because amyl nitrate significantly decreases systemic blood pressure and therefore blood flow to the fetus, use is contraindicated in pregnancy (per manufacturer).

2) Other options exist to treat cyanide exposure including sodium nitrite, sodium thiosulfate, and hydroxocobalamin.

7. Penicillamine (chelator)-Category D

In most cases, the benefits of short-term use probably outweigh the risk, especially when accounting for the health and prognosis of the mother.

Author: Bryan Hayes

美国急诊临床必知200招

173. 解毒剂的安全性与妊娠

1.很多解毒剂在妊娠期的应用都没有经过足够的研究，被美国食品与药品监督管理局标记为妊娠危险分类'C'。但有几个解毒剂被定为'D'或'X'(禁忌的)。

2.乙醇(有毒的酒精)——分类 C

1)酒精注射对生育的影响还没有报导。乙醇可通过胎盘进入胎儿循环，在人身上有致畸作用。在妊娠中晚期作为解毒剂使用，短期治疗不会造成胎儿酒精综合征。在妊娠早期的应用有争议。

2)可替代(推荐)的解毒剂：甲吡唑

3.亚甲基兰(高铁血红蛋白血症)——分类 X

有证据显示经羊水穿刺给药可造成胎儿异常，但口服用药没有类似的不良后果。可能可以静脉用药。

4.劳拉西泮和地西泮(癫痫、神经毒剂)——分类 D

动物和人试验都发现有致畸作用，劳拉西泮和地西泮及它们的代谢物可通过人胎盘。

5.碘化钾(放射活性碘)——分类 D

碘可通过胎盘(可造成胎儿/新生儿甲状腺功能低下或甲状腺肿大。根据风险效益分析，可以用来防止由于暴露于放射碘而引起的甲状腺癌，需要注意的是使用的剂量和时间。

6.亚硝酸异戊酯(氰化物)——分类 C(厂商建议禁用)

1)还没有动物的繁殖试验。但由于亚硝酸异戊酯会明显地降低血压，减少胎儿血流，因此妊娠期禁用(根据厂商建议)。

2)在治疗氰化物中毒时可有其他的选择：亚硝酸钠、硫代硫酸钠和羟钴胺。

7.青霉胺(螯合剂)——分类 D

在很多情况下，特别是考虑到母亲的健康和预后，短期的效益要超过风险。

参考文献：

Lexi-Comp Online, Lexi-Drugs Online, Hudson, Ohio: Lexi-Comp, Inc.; February 14, 2013.

作者：Bryan Hayes

药物中毒

411

174. Dexmedetomidine for Cocaine Induced Sympathomimetic Activity?

1. Cocaine toxicity is characterized by the sympathomimetic toxidrome: tachycardia, hypertension, hyperpyrexia, diaphoresis as well as sodium channel blocking effects that can cause local anesthesia topically, QRS widening and even seizure.

2. Usual treatment for a cocaine toxic patient is benzodiazepines and cooling. Be wary of end organ damage, trauma and seizures.

3. There was a recent study that looked at dexmedetomidine to treat the sympathomimetic effects. Placebo-controlled trial used cocaine-addicted volunteer and applied intranasal cocaine. Measuring skin sympathetic nerve activity and skin vascular resistance.

4. This highlights the incredible physiologic mechanism of catecholamine release from the CNS with cocaine.

Author: Fermin Barrueto

174. 右美托咪定治疗
可卡因导致的拟交感神经活性

1. 可卡因中毒的特点是拟交感神经中毒症状：心动过速、高血压、高热、大汗、由钠离子通道阻断作用产生的局部麻醉作用、QRS 波增宽和癫痫。

2. 对于可卡因中毒患者的常规治疗包括苯二氮䓬类药物和降温，要警惕脏器衰竭、外伤和癫痫。

3. 一项最近发表的研究使用右美托咪定治疗拟交感神经反应，这个安慰剂对照试验给可卡因成瘾自愿者鼻内给予可卡因，测量皮肤交感神经活性和皮肤血管阻力。

4. 试验结果进一步证实了可卡因促使中枢神经系统释放儿茶酚胺的生理机制。

参考文献：

Dexmedetomidine as a novel countermeasure for cocaine-induced central sympathoexcitation in cocaine-addicted humans. Kontak AC, Victor RG, Vongpatanasin W. Hypertension. 2013 Feb; 61 (2)：388 – 394

作者：**Fermin Barrueto**

药
物
中
毒

175. Ricin-of course

1. On 4/16/2013, the United States Capitol Police (USCP) was notified by the Senate mail handling facility that it received an envelope containing a white granular substance. The envelope was immediately quarantined by the facility's personnel and USCP HAZMAT responded to the scene. Preliminary tests indicate the substance found was Ricin.

2. A few notes about ricin seems appropriate:

1) Easy to make from castor bean though heat labile.

2) No antidote, though Fab like digibind is in development.

3) Granule size of the grain of sand can kill.

4) Inhalation, IM, IV all effective.

5) After immediate exposure likely no symptoms.

6) Vomiting and diarrhea initially, acute lung injury and death in 3 − 5 days.

Author: Fermin Barrueto

175. 蓖麻毒素
（美国国会大厦 4 月 6 日事件的启示）

1. 2013 年 4 月 16 日，美国参议院邮件处理机构向美国国会大厦警察（USCP）报告，他们收到一个信封，里面有白色颗粒状物质。负责人员将信封立即隔离，USCP危险品控制局马上到了现场。初步测试表明，该物质是蓖麻毒素。

2. 对蓖麻毒素的认识有如下几点

1）热不稳定，容易从蓖麻子中提取。

2）没有解药，与地高辛特异性抗体（digibind）类似的特异性抗体片段正在研发中。

3）一粒沙子大小的剂量就可致死。

4）吸入、肌肉注射、静脉注射有同样效果。

5）接触后可能不会马上出现症状。

6）以呕吐和腹泻起病，在 3 ~ 5 天内出现急性肺损伤以至死亡。

参考文献：

CDC website：http：//www.bt.cdc.gov/agent/ricin

作者：**Fermin Barrueto**

药物中毒

415

176. DKA Deaths Due to 2nd Generation Antipsychotics

1. Hyperglycemia in the setting of antipsychotic use has been reported mostly with olanzapine (Zyprexa) but does occur with other antipsychotics. A recent study from the NYC medical examiner's office details 17 deaths of DKA due to antipsychotics and found that (from highest to lowest incidence) quetiapine > olanzapine > risperidone were the atypical antipsychotics found with these deaths.

2. Remember hyperglycemia occurs with patients on antipsychotics and can lead to hyperglycemia hyperosmolar coma or DKA. Both can be lethal.

Author: FerminBarrueto

176. 第二代抗精神病药导致的
糖尿病酮症酸致死

1. 服用抗精神病药产生的高血糖多与奥氮平有关，但也可由其他抗精神病药造成。最近一篇来自纽约医学检察官办公室的文章详细报道了 17 例因抗精神病药导致的死亡，发现这些死亡都与非特异性抗精神病药有关，包括(按频率顺序)喹硫平、奥氮平和利培酮。

2. 服用抗精神病药的患者可出现高血糖，导致高血糖高渗性昏迷或糖尿病酮症酸中毒。二者均可导致死亡。

参考文献：

Fatal Diabetic Ketoacidosis and Antipsychotic Medication.

Ely SF, Neitzel AR, Gill JR.

J Forensic Sci. 2012 Dec 27. doi: 10. 1111/1556 – 4029. 12044.

作者：**FerminBarrueto**

药物中毒

药物与治疗
Pharmacology and Therapeutics

177. 10 New Drugs and Devices from 2011—2012 That Might Change Your EM Practice

1. Xarelto® (rivaroxaban)-a Factor Xa inhibitor for treating venous thromboembolic disease (VTE)

For prophylaxis of deep vein thrombosis (DVT) in adults undergoing hip and knee replacement surgery; for stroke prophylaxis in patients with non-valvular atrial fibrillation; on November 2, 2012, for the treatment of patients with DVT and PE and for long-term treatment to prevent recurrence.

2. Eliquis® (apixaban) -another direct factor Xa inhibitor

for reducing the risk of stroke and systemic embolism in patients with atrial fibrillation that is not caused by a heart valve problem.

3. Brilinta® (ticagrelor)-an antiplatelet agent

for secondary prevention of stent thrombosis, cardiovascular death, and heart attack in patients with acute coronary syndrome (ACS).

4. Tudorza® (aclidinium bromide)-an inhalational anticholinergic agent for COPD / emphysema.

Twice-daily dosing. Ipratropium bromide (Atrovent®), four-time-daily dosing and tiotropium (Spiriva®) once-daily.

5. Sklice® (ivermectin)-topical treatment of head lice infestation

One time treatment.

6. Subsys® (fentanyl sublingual spray formulation for breakthrough cancer pain)

Healthcare professionals who prescribe Subsys® on an outpatient basis must first enroll in the Transmucosal Immediate Release Fentanyl Risk Evaluation and Mitigation Strategy.

7. Dificid® (fidaxomicin)-antibiotic specific for treatment of Clostridium difficile similar efficacy to vancomycin.

8. Rectiv® (nitroglycerin ointment 0.4%)-topical therapy for anal

The recommended dosage is one inch of ointment (375 mg of ointment equivalent to 1.5 mg of nitroglycerin) applied intra-anally every 12 hours up to three weeks.

9. Auvi-Q®-a talking dispenser of epinephrine/adrenaline

Auvi-Q® is an epinephrine auto-injector that is easy to carry and "talks" to you how to use it.

10. Zio-Patch®-a device for monitoring dysrhythmias in outpatients

The Zio® Patch is a single-use, noninvasive waterproof continuous monitoring patch worn on the chest that provides continuous monitoring for up to 14 days.

Author: Feng Xiao (肖锋)

药
物
与
治
疗

177. 2011—2012 年出现的 10 种新药或新仪器

1. 拜瑞妥®（利伐沙班）——Xa 因子抑制药，治疗静脉血栓栓塞症（VTE）。

可预防成人髋关节和膝关节置换术后深静脉血栓（DVT）形成；预防非瓣膜性房颤患者脑卒中的发生。2012 年 11 月 2 日，FDA 批准新增适应证，DVT 和肺动脉栓塞的治疗和长期复发预防。

2. Eliquis®（阿哌沙班）——另一个直接 Xa 因子抑制药。

可减少非心脏瓣膜问题引起的心房颤动导致脑卒中和全身性栓塞的风险。

3. Brilinta®（替卡格雷）——一种抗血小板药，急性冠脉综合征（ACS）患者的支架内血栓形成、心血管死亡和心肌梗死的二级预防。

4. Tudorza®（阿地溴铵）——用于治疗 COPD/肺气肿的吸入性抗胆碱能制剂，每日两次。异丙托溴铵（爱喘乐®），每日四次；噻托溴铵（思力华®）每日一次。

5. Sklice®（伊维菌素）——外用治疗头虱。

一次性治疗。

6. SUBSYS®（芬太尼舌下喷雾制剂控制癌症疼痛）。

门诊医生开 SUBSYS® 的处方权必须先加入"共享经黏膜吸收即时释放芬太尼风险控制和降低评估系统"（TIRFREMS）。

7. Dificid®（非达霉素）——治疗艰难梭菌的特异性抗生素。

与万古霉素有相似的疗效。

8. fissure Rectiv®（硝酸甘油软膏 0.4%）——外用治疗肛裂。

每次挤出 2.54 cm 的药膏，将其置入（375 毫克，相当于 1.5 毫克硝酸甘油软膏）肛门内，每 12 小时一次，可连用三个星期。

9. Auvi-Q®－带语音提示的肾上腺素注射器。

Auvi-Q® 是一种肾上腺素自动注射器，很容易携带并可指示你如何使用它。

10. 齐奥粘片®－一种在院外监测心律失常的设备。

齐奥粘片® 是一次性使用的非侵入性防水连续心电监测粘片。它戴在胸前，可提供长达 14 天的连续心电监测。

参考文献：

Joe Lex. New Drugs and Devices from 2011 – 2012 That Might Change Your Practice http：// www. emedhome. com/features_archive_detail. cfm

药
物
与
治
疗

423

178. Cross-reactivity Between Sulfonamide Antimicrobials and Non-Antimicrobials

1. Patients frequently report having a sulfa allergy. In most cases, the allergic reaction was secondary to a sulfonamide antimicrobial agent, such as sulfamethoxazole-trimethoprim.

2. The question is: Can I use furosemide (or other non-antimicrobial agents containing a sulfa component)?

3. There is minimal evidence of cross-reactivity between sulfonamide antimicrobials and non-antimicrobials.

4. Despite this, the U. S. FDA-approved product information for many non-antimicrobial sulfonamide drugs contains warnings concerning possible cross-reactions.

5. Bottom line: If a patient had a true IgE-mediated anaphylactic reaction to a sulfonamide antimicrobial, it may be best to avoid other sulfa-related medications (use ethacrynic acid if a loop diuretic is needed). Otherwise, the available literature does not support cross-reactivity between sulfonamide antimicrobials and non-antimicrobials.

Author: Bryan Hayes

178. 磺胺类抗生素和
非抗生素之间的交叉反应

1.经常会有患者对磺胺过敏,多数情况下是对磺胺类抗生素有过敏反应,如磺胺甲基异恶唑 – 甲氧苄氨嘧啶(复方新诺明)。

2.问题是我可以用速尿(或其他非抗生素类磺胺制剂)吗?

3.几乎没有证据证实磺胺类的抗生素和非抗生素之间有交叉反应。

4.尽管如此,在美国食品与药品监督管理局批准的非抗生素磺胺类药品说明书中,仍有交叉反应危险的警示。

5.结论:如果患者对磺胺类抗生素确实有 IgE 导致的过敏反应,最好避免任何其他含磺胺类的药物(如必须用袢利尿药可用依他尼酸代替)。然而,到目前为止还没有证据证实磺胺类抗生素和非抗生素之间有交叉反应。

参考文献:

Strom BL, et al. Absence of cross-reactivity between sulfonamide antibiotics and sulfonamide non-antibiotics. N Engl J Med 2003;349(17):1628 – 1635.

Hemstreet BA, et al. Sulfonamide allergies and outcomes related to use of potentially cross-reactive drugs in hospitalized patients. Pharmacother 2006;26(4):551 – 557.

Lee AG, et al. Presumed "sulfa allergy" in patients with intracranial hypertension treated with acetazolamide or furosemide:cross-reactivity, myth or reality? Am J Ophthalmol 2004;138(1):114 – 118.

Johnson KK, et al. Sulfonamide cross-reactivity:fact or fiction? Ann Pharmacother 2005;39(2):290 – 301.

作者:**Bryan Hayes**

药
物
与
治
疗

179. Intravenous Phenergan

If you are still using IV Phenergan, you need to be aware of the necrotic effect that occurs if it infiltrates. EDs have even removed it from their drug dispensing machines. It appears to be the drug and not the diluent. Mechanism is not completely understood. Below is a picture the plaintiff attorney will use about this well known adverse effect. If so many alternatives for IV antiemetic it is wise to reconsider IV Phenergan.

1) Why give it IM? Absorption rate is faster than SQ infiltration though theoretically could still cause necrosis.

2) Is it only infiltration? Gangrene has occurred with inadvertent intra-arterial injection, SQ infiltration and even regular IV administration.

3) Mechanism? Appears to be the drug and not diluent, diluting down the concentration as well as decreasing dose appears to help if you are going to give it IV.

Author: Fermin Barrueto

179. 静脉注射非那根

　　如果你还在使用静脉注射非那根,你必须考虑如果它发生外渗将导致浸润性坏死。急诊科已经将它从常备药柜里剔除。这似乎是药物本身的原因而与稀释剂无关,其机制尚未完全了解。本文插图是原告律师用来证实这个已是众所周知的副作用。在有这么多静脉止呕药作为选择的情况下,重新考虑静脉注射非那根将是一种明智的做法。

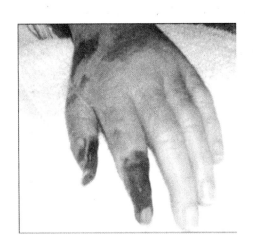

　　1)为什么通过肌肉注射给药? 吸收率要比皮下渗透快,虽然理论上仍然可以引起坏死。
　　2)坏死只发生在渗出后吗? 坏死还发生在不慎动脉内注射、皮下注射,甚至常规静脉给药。
　　3)机制? 这似乎是药物本身的问题而与稀释剂无关,如果要静脉给药,稀释浓度以及减小剂量似乎有所帮助。

作者:Fermin Barrueto

180. Intranasal fentanyl

1. Who: Young, otherwise healthy pediatric patients undergoing minor procedures (laceration repair, fracture reduction/splinting, etc...).

2. What: Fentanyl (2 mcg/kg).

3. When: 5 minutes pre-procedure.

4. Where: Intranasal.

5. Why: More effective than PO, less invasive than IV while being equally efficacious.

6. How: Use an atomizer, splitting the dose between each nostril.

Author: Mimi Lu

180. 鼻内用芬太尼

1. 应用对象：年轻，原本健康的需要行小手术（裂伤修补术、骨折复位/夹板等）的小儿患者。

2. 用什么：芬太尼（2 mg/kg）。

3. 什么时间用：操作前 5 分钟。

4. 用药途经：鼻内。

5. 为什么？ 比口服更有效，比静脉给药创伤小但有同样效果。

6. 如何用？ 使用雾化器，将剂量分配到每个鼻孔。

参考文献：

1）Use of Intranasal Fentanyl for the Relief of Pediatric Orthopedic Trauma Pain, Mary Saunders, MD Academic Emergency Medicine 2010, 17：1155 – 1161.

2）A Randomized Controlled Trial Comparing Intranasal Fentanyl to Intravenous Morphine for Managing Acute Pain in children in the Emergency Department, Meredith Borland, MBBS, FACEM, Annals of Emergency Medicine, March 2007, Vol. 49, No. 3, 335 – 340

3）The Implementation of Intranasal Fentanyl for Children in a Mixed Adult and Pediatric Emergency Department Reduces time to analgesic Administration, Anna Holdgate, MBBS, Academic Emergency Medicine 2010, 17：214 – 217.

作者：**Mimi Lu**

药物与治疗

429

181. Sotalol-watch out, review med list

1. When reviewing a patient's medication list, there are always some that should catch your eyes. Digoxin is one since we can measure it, has a low therapeutic index and elimination is effected when renal function is diminished. Another drug that should catch your eyes is SOTALOL. Renally cleared and affected by even a minimally lower than normal magnesium. The toxic effect even at therapeutic levels is torsades de pointes.

2. One study, in a 736 bed hospital, showed 89% of patients prescribed sotalol were on an inappropriate dose due to renal function and an odds ratio of 3.7 increased re-admission rate at 6 months for the patients on the inappropriate dose of sotalol.

3. We can catch this in the ED. Involve your pharmacist, ED pharmacist or local toxicologist for dosing calculations.

Author: Fermin Barrueto

181. 索他洛尔——小心，要检查药单

1. 审查患者的用药清单时，总会有一些药物吸引你的眼球。地高辛是其中之一。它的浓度可测，治疗指数低，当肾功能减退时，它的排出会受影响。应该抓住你眼球的另一种药物是索他洛尔，它是由肾脏清除的，稍微低于正常水平的镁也会影响其作用。即使在治疗水平，其毒性作用也可致尖端扭转型室性心动过速。

2. 一项来自于拥有 736 张病床医院的研究显示，有 89% 的患者服用与肾功能不相符剂量的索他洛尔；服用不适当剂量的索他洛尔会使患者在 6 个月内的再住院率增加 3.7 倍。

3. 我们可以在急诊科发现这一问题。在确定剂量时，可征求你的药剂师、急诊科的药剂师或当地毒理学中心的意见。

参考文献：

Finks SW, Rogers KC, Manguso AH. Assessment of sotalol prescribing in a community hospital: opportunities for clinical pharmacist involvement [J]. Int J Pharm Pract. 2011 Aug; 19 (4): 281 –286.

作者：Fermin Barrueto

药物与治疗

182. Opioid Induced Hyperalgesia

1. Opioid analgesia can actually INCREASE sensitivity to pain in some cases.

2. The exact cause is unclear, but may be due to up-regulation of NDMA receptors in spinal cord dorsal horn neurons.

3. Pain tends to be DIFFERENT and DIFFUSE from the underlying condition for which the narcotics were prescribed.

4. Switching from shorter acting opiates to methadone may be effective, as it is a weak NDMA antagonist and has only partial cross tolerance with other opioids.

Author: Ellen Lemkin

美
国
急
诊
临
床
必
知
200
招

182. 阿片类镇痛药导致的疼痛敏感性增加

1. 在某些情况下，阿片类镇痛药实际上可以增加对疼痛的敏感性。

2. 虽然确切原因尚不清楚，但可能是由于脊髓后角神经元 NDMA 受体上调。

3. 疼痛往往是弥漫性疼痛片与阿片药治疗的疼痛性质不同。

4. 从短效阿片类转成美沙酮可能会是有效的，因为它是一种弱的 NDMA 阻断药，与其他类阿片药物只有部分交叉耐药性。

参考文献：

Gussow, L. Toxicology Rounds. When Opioids Increase Pain. Emergency Medicine News Feb 2013. 35(2): 6.

作者：**Ellen Lemkin**

药物与治疗

183. 2012 Beers Criteria update from the American Geriatrics Society?

1. The American Geriatrics Society updated Beers Criteria for potentially inappropriate medication use in older adults is now available.

2. The update differs in several ways from the 2003 edition. Medications that are no longer available have been removed, and drugs introduced since 2003 have been added. Research on drugs included in earlier versions has been updated and new information is provided about appropriate prescribing of medications for an expanded list of common geriatric conditions.

3. Here is an abbreviated list of medications/classes on the list that we may use in the ED. Use caution.

1) Anticholinergics.

2) Nitrofurantoin.

3) Clonidine.

4) Antidysrhythmics.

5) Digoxin.

6) Antipsychotics.

7) Benzodiazepines.

8) Insulin.

9) Metoclopramide.

10) NSAIDs.

Author: Bryan Hayes

183. 2012 年美国老年病学会新的 Beers 标准

1. 美国老年病学会发表了新一版的 Beers 标准，旨在减少老年人潜在的用药不适。

2. 新标准与 2003 版比较有几方面的不同。不再使用的药物被剔除，同时增加了 2003 年以后的新药。更新了包括在先前版本中的药物的研究进展，丰富了老年常见病药物种类，并提供了有关正确使用它们的信息。

3. 这是一个简化的在急诊科常用的药物/药物种类的目录，（在老年患者中）要小心应用。

1）抗胆碱能药；

2）呋喃妥因；

3）可乐定；

4）抗心律失常药；

5）地高辛；

6）抗精神病药；

7）镇静催眠药；

8）胰岛素；

9）胃复安；

10）非甾体类抗炎药。

参考文献：

The American Geriatrics Society 2012 Beers Criteria Update Expert Panel. American Geriatrics Society Updated Beers Criteria for Potentially Inappropriate Medication Use in Older Adults. J Am Geriatr Soc 2012；60（4）：616－631.

作者：Bryan Hayes

药物与治疗

435

184. Emergency Hospitalizations for ADEs in Older Americans

1. A recent article estimated 100, 000 emergency hospitalizations for adverse drug events in U. S. adults 65 years of age or older each year. Nearly half of these hospitalizations were among adults ≥80 years old and two-thirds were due to unintentional overdoses.

2. Four medications or medication classes were implicated alone or in combination in 67% of hospitalizations:

1) Warfarin (33.3%).

2) Insulins (13.9%).

3) Oral antiplatelet agents (13.3%).

4) Oral hypoglycemic agents (10.7%).

3. Opioids were #5. Digoxin was #7 and resulted in the highest percentage of hospitalizations per ED visit at 80%.

Author: Bryan Hayes

184. 美国老年人因药物不良反应 而紧急入院的情况

1. 一篇新的文章预测美国每年有 10 万 65 岁及以上的患者因药物的不良反应而入院，其中接近二分之一的入院患者年龄超过 80 岁，而三分之二是因为无意的服药过量。

2. 下面四种药的单独或合用占这些住院患者的 67% 。

1) 华法林(33.3%)。

2) 胰岛素(13.9%)。

3) 口服抗血小板药(13.3%)。

4) 口服降糖药(10.7%)。

3. 阿片类药物名列第五。地高辛列第七，但在急诊就诊患者中其住院率是最高的(80%)。

参考文献：

Budnitz DS, et al. Emergency hospitalizations for adverse drug events in older Americans. N Engl J Med 2011; 365: 2002 – 2012.

作者：**Bryan Hayes**

药物与治疗

185. Nicardipine vs Labetalol for Blood Pressure Management in the ED

1. A recent randomized trial compared nicardipine as a continuous infusion to labetalol boluses to determine which one was more effective at lowering blood pressure to a target range within 30 minutes.

2. Median initial SBP for the 226 patients was 212 mm Hg. Within 30 minutes, nicardipine patients more often reached target range than labetalol (91.7 vs. 82.5% , P =0.039). Of 6 BP measures (taken every 5 minutes) during the study period, nicardipine patients had higher rates of five and six instances within target range than labetalol (47.3% vs. 32.8% , $P = 0.026$).

3. What this means: Nicardipine is a reasonable choice for patients needing acute lowering of blood pressure (e. g. , ischemic stroke with tPa). Nicardipine seems to achieve faster and smoother lowering of blood pressure than labetalol therapy with less blood pressure readings outside the target range.

Author: Bryan Hayes

185. 尼卡地平和拉贝洛尔在急诊科高血压处理中的作用

1. 一项新的随机临床试验对持续静脉点滴尼卡地平和静脉缓推拉贝洛尔在降压作用进行了比较,以确定谁能在 30 分钟内将血压控制在理想范围内。

2. 226 个患者的平均初始收缩压(SBP)为 212 mmHg。在 30 分钟内,与拉贝洛尔组(82.5%)相比,更多的接受尼卡地平(91.7%,$P = 0.039$)的患者达到了理想目标。在试验时间内的 6 次血压测定(1 次/5 min)中,尼卡地平组患者有达到理想范围的频率要明显高于拉贝洛尔组患者(47.3% vs. 32.8%,$P = 0.026$)。

3. 这意味着在需要紧急降压时(如缺血性脑梗死需要 tPA 治疗),尼卡地平比拉贝洛尔能更快更平稳地使血压降至理想值范围内。

参考文献:

Peacock WF, Varon J, Baumann BM, et al. CLUE: a randomized comparative effectiveness trial of IV nicardipine versus labetalol use in the emergency department. Crit Care 2011; 15(3): R157. Epub 2011 Jun 27.

作者: **Bryan Hayes**

186. ACE inhibitor induced angioedema

1. Angioedema is induced by elevated levels of bradykinin.

2. Bradykinin is noramlly degraded by angiotensin-1 converting enzyme and several other enzymes (including aminipeptidase-P).

3. A deficiency in aminopeptidase-P likely leads to ACEI induced angioedema.

4. Treatment typically starts with discontinuing ACE inhibitors, administering H1 and H2 antagonists, and corticosteroids (all Class indeterminate).

5. Another consideration may be FFP 10 – 15 ml/kg IV or the off label use of icatibant (both Class II recommendations).

6. Icatibant inhibits the bradykin B2 receptor. It is a sythetic decapeptide structurally similar to bradykin.

7. Icatibant has been effective in case reports and case series in ACEI induced angioedema. There is a prospective, double blind randomized placebo controlled trial underway.

Author: Ellen Lemkin

美
国
急
诊
临
床
必
知
200
招

186. 血管紧张素转化酶抑制剂
导致的血管性水肿

1. 血管性水肿是由缓激肽的升高造成的。

2. 缓激肽在正常情况下是由血管紧张素 - 1 转化酶和其他几种酶(如氨基酸肽酶 - P)降解的。

3. 氨基酸肽酶缺乏很可能导致 ACEI 性血管性水肿。

4. 治疗主要是停止 ACEI 的继续使用,给 H1 和 H2 拮抗药及激素(疗效级别不定)。

5. 另外可考虑静脉应用新鲜冰冻血浆(fresh frozen plasma,FFP)10 ~ 15 mL/kg 或的药品核准标示外使用艾替班特(两者都是二类推荐药)。

6. 艾替班特可抑制缓激肽 B2 受体,是在结构上与缓激肽相似的十肽。

7. 艾替班特在 ACEI 导致的血管性水肿中的效果已有个例和系列病例报道,现在正在进行一项前瞻性的双盲随机对照剂控制的临床试验。

参考文献:

Wilerson G. Angioedema in the Emergency Department:An evidence-based review. Emergency Medicine Practice,Nov 2012.

作者:**Ellen Lemkin**

药物与治疗

441

187. Prevention of Contrast-Induced Nephropathy

1. There have been many attempts to reduce the incidence of contrast-induced nephropathy.

2. Mechanism usually centers around antioxidant properties or free radical scavengers that prevent the acute kidney injury that may result after intravenous contrast.

3. IV Fluid hydration, sodium bicarbonate and acetylcysteine have been studied with only some evidence.

4. There is also some controversial data that is beginning to surface regarding the use of atorvastatin with a recent article in Circulation 2012 that showed high dose atorvastatin (80 mg) 24 hrs prior to angiography prevented contrast-induced acute kidney injury in patients with mild to medium risk.

Author: FerminBarrueto

187. 阿托伐他汀(立普妥)
与造影剂肾病的预防

1. 减少造影剂肾病的发生有很多措施。

2. 机制通常是基于防止静脉造影剂造成的急性肾损伤而使用抗氧化药及游离基清除药。

3. 静脉输液、碳酸氢钠和乙酰半胱氨酸已被临床应用,虽然疗效还没有足够的证据。

4. 最近有一些资料开始报道阿托伐他汀(立普妥)的作用。在 2012 年《循环》杂志中有一篇文章显示,血管造影前 24 小时给予轻中度患者高剂量(80 mg)的阿托伐他汀(立普妥),可以防止造影剂导致的急性肾损伤。

参考文献:

http://circ.ahajournals.org/content/126/25/3008

作者:FerminBarrueto

药
物
与
治
疗

443

188. Levetiracetam（Keppra）
for Status Epileptics

1. Although Keppra has been used more frequently in clinical practice, there is little evidence for its use in status epilepticus.

2. It has a wide spectrum of action and few drug interactions.

3. Initially, case series appeared to be highly successful in terminating seizures as an add-on agent.

4. A review of 2 prospective studies found efficacies of 44% as an add- on agent, and 75% as a primary agent. The studies had markedly different populations.

5. In a retrospective study, the treatment failure rates were 3X higher than that of intravenous valproic acid as an add-on agent in terminating status epilepticus.

6. Therefore, although it is used frequently, the evidence for use is limited and inconclusive in terminating status epilepticus.

Author：Ellen Lemkin

美
国
急
诊
临
床
必
知
200
招

188. 左乙拉西坦在癫痫持续状态中的应用

1. 虽然左乙拉西坦在临床实践中已被广泛应用,但它在癫痫持续状态中应用的资料有限。

2. 它的作用广泛并很少有药物之间的反应。

3. 系列病例报告显示它作为一种终止癫痫的辅助药的效果是非常理想的。

4. 一篇对两个前瞻性研究文献的综述发现,左乙拉西坦作为辅助药的效果为44%,作为一线药的效果为75%。这些研究的研究人群中有明显差别。

5. 在一个回顾性报告中,它作为终止癫痫持续状态辅助药的治疗失败率是丙戊酸钠的3倍。

6. 因此,虽然它应用广泛,但尚无明确和足够证据支持它在治疗癫痫持续状态中的应用。

参考文献:

Trinka E. What is the evidence to use new intravenous AED in status epilepticus? Epilepsia 2011 52(Suppl 8):35 – 8.

Zelano J, Kumlien E. Levetiracetam as alternative stage two antiepileptic drug in status epilepticus: A systematic review. Seizure 2012. 21:233 – 6.

作者:**Ellen Lemkin**

药物与治疗

189. Wait—the creatinine is what?

1. General Information:

The two main units used by medical laboratories are "conventional (used in the US) and SI (used by most other countries)."

2. Pearls to know:

1) For monovalent ions (i. e. Na^+, Cl^-)—mEq/L = mmol/L (135 mEq = 135 mmol/L).

2) For divalent ions (i. e. ionized Ca^{2+}, Mg^{2+})—mEq/2 = mmol (Mg^2 + of 2 mEq/L = 1 mmol/L).

3) Creatinine—Multiply conventional untis by 88 (1 mg/dL = 88 mmol/L).

4) Glucose—Multiply SI units by 18 (4 mmol/L = 72 mg/dL).

5) Hemoglobin—Multiply conventional units by 10 (14 g/dL = 140 g/L).

3. Relevance to the EM Physician

These tips will help you convert labs to familiar values when reading medical literature, when working in another country, or when working with international colleagues.

Author: Andrea Tenner

189. 等一等！肌酐是多少？
（传统和国际单位的转换）

1. 简介

医学文献采用两个主要单位，传统的（用于美国）和国际的（SI，用于许多其他国家）。

2. 要记住的是

1）单价离子（Na^+，Cl^-）：mEq/L = mmol/L（135 mEq = 135 mmol/L）。

2）双价离子（离子化的 Ca^{2+}，Mg^{2+}）：mEq/2 = mmol 如 Mg^{2+} 浓度：2 mEg/L = 1 mmol/L。

3）肌酐：传统单位 ×88（1 mg/dl = 88 mmol/L）。

4）血糖：SI 单位 ×18（4 mmol/L = 72 mg/dl）。

5）血红蛋白：传统单位 ×10（14 g/dl = 140 g/L）。

3. 对急诊医生的意义

当阅读文献、在另外一个国家工作或与国际同行共事时，这些秘诀将会帮助你把实验室结果转成你所熟悉的单位。

参考文献：

Iverson C, Christiansen S, Flanagin A, et al. AMA Manual of Style: A Guide for Authors and Editors. 10th ed. New York, NY: Oxford University Press; 2007.

Ruschin, H and LoRusso J. Normal Values for Selected Blood and Urine Tests. Wiley. http://www.wiley.com/college/bio/tortora366927/resources/faculty/pdf/appb.pdf

作者：Andrea Tenner

药物与治疗

儿科急诊
Pediatrics

190. Pediatric Emergency Care Guidelines

1. General Information:

An estimated 70 children in the world die every 5 minutes—99% of these deaths are from developing countries, half in Sub-Saharan Africa, and two-thirds from preventable or easily treatable causes.

2. Area of the world affected:

One study examining the quality of hospital emergency care of 131 children in 21 hospitals in 7 developing countries found:

1)66% of hospitals did not have adequate triage; 41% of patients had inadequate initial assessment.

2)44% received inappropriate treatment and 30% had insufficient monitoring.

3)Frequent essential drugs, laboratory and radiology services supply outages.

4)Staffing and knowledge shortages for medical and nursing personnel.

3. Bottom Line

The IFEM International Standards for Emergency Care of Children provide an excellent resource for both clinicians and hospital managers in developing countries.

Author: Andrea Tenner

190. 国际儿科急诊医疗指南

1. 一般资料

世界上大概每5分钟会有70名儿童死亡，99%的死亡发生在发展中国家，一半在撒哈拉以南的非洲地区，其中三分之二死于可预防或可治疗的疾病。

2. 受影响的国际地区

对7个发展中国家21家医院的131名儿童在急诊的治疗质量研究发现：

1）66%的医院没有合理的分诊，41%的患者没有进行合理的初步评估；

2）44%的患者接受了不恰当的治疗，30%没有足够的监测；

3）基本药物供应、实验室和放射学检查中断；

4）医护人员配备和知识的短缺。

3. 要点

国际急诊医学联合会（IFEM）发表的儿童紧急医疗国际标准为发展中国家的医生和医院管理者提供了一个很好的参考。

参考文献：

Lozano R, Wang H, Foreman KJ, Rajaratnam JK, Naghavi M, Marcus JR, et al. Progress towards Millennium Development Goals 4 and 5 on maternal and child mortality: an updated systematic analysis. Lancet 2011; 378(9797): 1139 – 1165.

You D, Jones G, Hill K, Wardlaw T, Chopra M. Levels and trends in child mortality, 1990 – 2009. Lancet 2010; 376(9745): 931 – 933.

Cheema B. International standards of care for children in emergency centres-do they apply to Africa? African Journal of Emergency Medicine (2013) 3, 50 – 51

Nolan T, Angos P, Cunha AJ, Muhe L, Qazi S, Simoes EA, Tamburlini G, Weber M, Pierce NF. Quality of hospital care for seriously ill children in less-developed countries. Lancet 2001 Jan 13; 357(9250): 106 – 110.

International Standards for Emergency Care of Children in Emergency Departments. Full Document Available from: http://www.ifem.cc/Resources/PoliciesandGuidelines.aspx

作者：**Andrea Tenner**

儿科急诊

191. Otitis Media (2013 AAP AOM Guidelines UPDATES)

AAP released a new clinical practice guideline for diagnosis and management of acute otitis media (AOM).

Key Action Statements:

1. Diagnosis: presence of middle ear effusion and:

1) moderate to severe bulging of tympanic membrane (TM) or new otorrhea or.

2) mild bulging of TM and recent ear pain or intense erythema of TM.

2. Treatment options

1) Severe unilateral or bilateral AOM (>6 months): give antibiotics. Severe AOM is defined as fever >102.2 (39 C), moderate/severe otalgia, or symptoms >48 h.

2) Nonsevere unilateral AOM (6 – 23 months): Advise the parents to consider a period of close observation and follow up (24 – 72 h). If the child's clinical status deteriorates, give antibiotics.

3) Nonsevere bilateral AOM (6 – 23 months): give antibiotics.

4) Nonsevere unilateral or bilateral AOM (> 24 months): Advise the parents to consider a period of close observation and follow up (24 – 72 h). If the child's clinical status deteriorates, give antibiotics.

Author: **Mimi Lu**

美国急诊临床必知200招

191. 2013 年美国儿科学会
急性中耳炎治疗指南更新

美国儿科学会最近公布了急性中耳炎(AOM)诊断和治疗的临床实践指南。
推荐方法概要如下：

1. 中耳炎的诊断：中耳有积液渗出且具有下列症状之一

1)中度到重度鼓膜隆突或新出现的耳漏

2)轻度鼓膜隆突和新的耳痛或鼓膜红肿

2. 治疗原则

1)严重的单侧或双侧 AOM(>6 个月)：抗生素治疗。严重 AOM 的定义为体温 >39℃，中度或重度耳痛，或症状超过 48 小时。

2)不严重的单侧 AOM (6~23 个月)：建议家长密切观察患者并在 24~72 小时内随诊。如患者临床状态恶化，应用抗生素治疗。

3)不严重的双侧 AOM 儿童(6~23 个月)：抗生素治疗。

4)不严重的单侧或双侧 AOM(>24 个月)：建议家长密切观察患者并在 24~72 小时内随诊。如患者临床状态恶化，应用抗生素治疗。

参考文献：

Pediatrics Vol. 131 No. 3 March 1, 2013

作者：**Mimi Lu**

儿科急诊

453

192. Drug-Induced Seizures
in Children and Adolescents

1. Seizures can be the presenting manifestation of acute poisoning in children.

2. A 3-year data set from the Toxicology Investigators Consortium (ToxIC) Case Registry identified 142 cases of drug-induced seizures in children < 18 years old. 75% were teenagers.

3. Antidepressants were most commonly associated with causing seizures, especially bupropion and citalopram. Diphenhydramine was also a commonly identified cause.

4. The authors conclude that clinicians managing teenagers presenting with seizures should have a high index of suspicion for intentional ingestion of antidepressants.

Author: Bryan Hayes

192. 儿童和青少年中药物引起的癫痫

1. 儿童急性中毒可以表现为癫痫发作。

2. 毒理学研究者协会(ToxIC)案例注册表中为期 3 年的数据显示，有 142 例低于 18 岁的儿童因药物中毒而出现癫痫发作，其中 75% 是青少年。

3. 最常见的与癫痫发作有关的药物是抗抑郁药，尤其是安非他酮和西酞普兰，苯海拉明也是一个常见的原因。

4. 作者认为，临床医生在处理青少年癫痫发作时应该高度警惕有可能的抗抑郁药中毒。

参考文献：

Finkelstein Y, et al. Drug-induced seizures in children and adolescsents presenting for emergency care: current and emerging trends. ClinToxicol 2013; 51(8): 761 – 766.

作者：**Bryan Hayes**

儿科急诊

193. The cough is keeping them awake all night!

1. How many times have you been frustrated in the peds ED when you have a child with a URI that has a significant night time cough and you feel like you have nothing to offer them for symptom control?

2. The parent is frustrated because the child is not sleeping which means they are not sleeping and they are looking at you for help.

3. We all know that OTC cough and cold medications are not helpful and may be harmful in children < 2 yrs old and should be used with caution in children < 6 yrs old.

4. So what can you do? You can recommend a course of HONEY at night. Of course this does not apply to children < 1 yr who are at increased risk of botulism.

5. A recent double-blind placebo-controlled trial published in Pediatrics in 2012 demonstrated reduced night time cough and subjective improved sleep quality in children age 1 − 5 who were given honey compared to placebo.

6. This study supports previous less rigorous publications that found honey was an effective remedy on cough in children. Mechanism for honey's beneficial effect on cough is unknown but possibly related to close anatomic relationship between sensory nerve fibers that initiate cough and gustatory nerve fibers that taste sweetness.

7. Of note, a recently published survey in Pediatric Emergency Care revealed that 2/3 of parents were unaware of the FDA guidelines regarding OTC cough and cold remedies in children!

8. After you recommend HONEY for night time cough, take an extra minute and educate your parents about the potential dangers of cough and cold medicines in small children!

Author: Danielle Devereaux

193. 咳嗽让他们彻夜难眠！

1. 你有多少次在儿科急诊为一个因上呼吸道感染而整夜咳嗽的患者纠结，你好像觉得在症状控制方面真是无能为力了？

2. 你很纠结，因为孩子不睡就意味着大人也睡不了。他们都需要你的帮助。

3. 我们都知道，有关咳嗽和感冒的非处方药没有多大帮助，甚至对 <2 岁的儿童是有害的，即使对 <6 岁的儿童也应慎用。

4. 那么，你能做些什么呢？你可以建议在晚上用一个疗程的蜂蜜。当然，这并不适用于 <1 岁的儿童，因为这可能增加肉毒杆菌感染的风险。

5. 最近发表在 2012 年《Pediatrics》杂志的一项双盲安慰剂对照试验证明，蜂蜜与安慰剂相比可减少 1~5 岁儿童的夜间咳嗽并改善睡眠质量。

6. 这项研究支持以前不太明确的有关蜂蜜是一种对小儿咳嗽有效的治疗措施的研究报告。蜂蜜有利于止咳的作用机制尚不清楚，但可能与主管咳嗽和甜味觉神经解剖关系相近有关。

7. 值得注意的是，最近公布的小儿急救护理调查显示，2/3 的家长对美国食品与药品监督管理局有关儿童咳嗽和感冒的非处方药的规定还不了解！

8. 当你推荐蜂蜜治疗夜间咳嗽时，要让父母知道小孩服用咳嗽和感冒药的潜在风险！

参考文献：

Cohen A, Rozen J, Kristal H, et al. Effect of honey on nocturnal cough and sleep quality: a double-blind, randomized, placebo-controlled study. Pediatrics. 2012; 130(2): 465 – 471.

Varney SM, et al. Survey in the emergency department of parents' understanding of cough and cold medication use in children younger than 2 years[J]. Pediatr Emerg Care. 2012; 28(9): 883 – 885.

作者：Danielle Devereaux

儿科急诊

194. The Life-Threatening Red Umbilical Cord

1. Should you be concerned about erythema around the umbilical stump?
Yes!

2. Often parents will bring their neonate to the ED with concerns about the umbilical cord and it is just a simple granuloma or normal detachment. But is it omphalitis???

3. Omphalitis incidence is low in developed countries, but that means it's easier, and no less catastrophic, to miss!

4. Omphalitis is a superficial cellulitis of the umbilical cord, but 10 – 16% progress to necrotizing fasciitis of the abdominal wall!!!

5. Always ADMIT and consider consulting surgery early in case of rapid progression...

6. Most often polymicrobial and should be treated with:

1) Anti-staphylococcal PCN, Vanc, & an Aminoglycoside.

2) Also consider adding Metronidazole or Clindamycin for anaerobic coverage.

3) Anti-pseudomonal coverage if toxic.

7. Should notice improvement within 12 – 24 hours, so if don't or begin to observe

1) Fever.

2) Induration.

3) Peau d'orange tissue.

4) Tenderness.

5) Violaceous discoloration.

6) Crepitace.

7) Increased erythema.

8) Systemic signs of toxicity/shock.

8. CONSULT SURERY for concern of necrotizing fasciitis which has a mortality rate of close to 60% !!!

194. 危及生命的脐带发红

1. 你应该小心脐带残端发红吗？

当然！

2. 家长往往会因担忧新生儿脐带问题而来急诊科就诊，它通常只是一个简单的肉芽肿或正常脱落，但它会是脐带炎吗？

3. 脐带炎在发达国家的发生率低，但是这意味着它更容易导致危险的误诊！

4. 脐带炎是脐带浅表的蜂窝织炎，但 10% ~ 16% 发展成腹壁坏死性筋膜炎！

5. 一定要住院治疗并在病情迅速恶化前请外科会诊。

6. 最常见的病因是多种微生物感染，应采取下列治疗措施：

1）金黄色葡萄球菌敏感的青霉素、万古霉素和氨基糖苷类。

2）对厌氧菌可考虑加用甲硝唑或克林霉素。

3）如患者中毒症状重，要用抗假单胞菌药。

7. 通常症状应在 12 ~ 24 小时内缓解，如果不好转，要开始观察是否存在如下症状和体征：

1）发热；

2）硬结；

3）橘皮样改变；

4）压痛；

5）变紫；

6）皮下捻发音；

7）红肿加重；

8）全身中毒反应或休克。

8. 对任何怀疑坏死性筋膜炎的患者，要请外科会诊，其死亡率接近 60%！

参考文献：

Pérez, David Vila, et al. "Prognostic Factors in Pediatric Sepsis Study, from the Spanish Society of Pediatric Intensive Care." The Pediatric Infectious Disease Journal (2013).

Sawin RS, Schaller RT, Tapper D. Early Recognition of Neonatal Abdominal Wall Necrotizing Fasciitis. American Journal of Surgery. May 1994; 167: 481 – 484.

Ulloa-Gutierrez R, Rodriguez-Calzada H, Quesada L, Arguello A. Is it Acute Omphalitis or Necrotizing Fasciitis? Report of Three Fatal Cases. Pediatric Emergency Care. Sept 2005; 21(9): 600 – 602.

作者：**Joey Scollan**

儿科急诊

195. Complications of Malaria Treatment in the Pediatric Population

1. Case Presentation:

You are working in an ED in Houston when a 2 year old girl presents with fever for one day and decreased po intake. On arrival her temp = 103, HR = 180, and RR = 50 SaO_2 = 100%. She was born in the US and is up to date on all of her vaccinations, but has just returned from a trip to Liberia where she was visiting her extended family and received multiple mosquito bites. Physical exam, CXR and urinalysis are otherwise unremarkable and you suspect malaria, based on her history. You start quinine IV while you are waiting for the smear when suddenly the child becomes unresponsive.

2. Clinical Question: What is the next investigation you should perform?

Answer: Rapid blood glucose!

3. This patient has at least 4 reasons to be hypoglycemic:

1) fasting (Kids can become hypoglycemic from fasting alone in ~24hrs).

2) infection (any infectious disease can cause it, esp in kids <3 yrs old).

3) malaria (thought to be due in part to increased consumption by parasite).

4) quinine (stimulates insulin release).

4. Bottom Line:

Kids can become hypoglycemic fast—check a blood glucose in all pre-pubertal sick children.

Author: Andrea Tenner

195. 治疗儿童疟疾患者的并发症

1. 病例介绍

当你在休斯敦的一个急诊科工作时，一个 2 岁的女孩因发热一天、进食减少就诊。当时她的体温为 39.4℃，心率为 180 次／分，呼吸频率为 50 次／分，血氧饱和度为 100%。她出生在美国，迄今为止已完成所有的疫苗接种。患者刚从利比里亚旅游回来，在那里被蚊虫叮咬多次，体检、胸部 X 光检查和尿检均正常，根据她的病史，你怀疑是疟疾。在等待涂抹片时，你开始静脉给予奎宁治疗，但发现孩子突然变得反应迟钝。

2. 临床问题：下一步你应该做什么？

答案：快速测血糖！

3. 这个患者血糖低至少有 4 个原因

1）空腹（孩子们可能在禁食 24 小时内发生低血糖）；

2）感染（任何传染病都可引起低血糖，尤其 3 岁以内小儿）；

3）疟疾（被认为部分原因是由于寄生虫消耗增加）；

4）奎宁（刺激胰岛素释放）。

4. 要点

孩子可以很快出现低血糖，对所有青春期前患重病的儿童要检查血糖。

参考文献：

Zijlmans WCWR et al. Glucose metabolism in children: influence of age, fasting, and infectious diseases. Metabolism Clinical and Experimental. 2009. 58: 1356 – 1365.

作者：**Andrea Tenner**

196. Pediatric UTI (Age 2 – 24 Months)

1. The diagnosis and treatment of pediatric urinary tract infections (UTIs) can be broken down into different age groups. The AAP has recently updated its recommendations for children age 2 – 24 months.

2. In ill-appearing febrile infants age 2 – 24 months, who require early initiation of antibiotics, clinicians should obtain urinalysis and urine culture by catheterization or suprapubic aspiration prior to administration of the first dose of antibiotics.

3. Key components of diagnosing a UTI include: urinalysis with the presence of pyuria (>10 WBCs per μL) and bacteriuria. The ultimate diagnosis relies on identification of >50, 000 CFUs per mL of a single urinary pathogen in culture.

4. Treatment of most UTIs in well appearing infants 2 – 24 months can be done with oral antibiotics for a course of 7 – 14 days. Common antibiotics used include: amoxicillin-clavulanate, trimethoprim-sulfamethoxazole, or cephalosporins (cefpodoxime, cefixime) based on local patterns of susceptibility.

5. Febrile infants should undergo renal and bladder ultrasound (RBUS) to evaluate the renal parenchyma and identify complications of UTI in children who are not responding to treatment within 48 hours.

6. Voiding cystourethrography (VCUG) to diagnose vesicoureteral reflux (VUR) as a cause of UTI should be only obtained in children with abnormal RBUS or with recurrent febrile UTIs.

Author: Lauren Rice

196. 小儿尿路感染

1. 儿童尿路感染(UTIS)的诊断和治疗分成不同的年龄组,美国儿科学会最近更新了对2~24个月儿童的建议。

2. 对看起来较重并发热需要尽快给抗生素的2~24个月的儿童,医生要在给抗生素前通过插尿管或耻骨上穿刺做尿常规和培养。

3. 诊断UTI的关键是:尿常规里有脓尿(超过10个WBC)和菌尿。确诊依赖于培养中有超过50 000 CFU/mL的单一尿致病菌。

4. 对看起来病情不重的2~24个月的儿童可用7~14天的口服抗生素,常用的抗生素包括:奥格门汀,甲氧苄氨嘧啶-磺胺甲基异恶唑或头孢菌素类(头孢泊肟,头孢克肟),要根据当地的抗菌谱选择。

5. 发热的患儿要做肾脏和膀胱超声检查(RBUS),以检查肾实质和发现48小时内对治疗无反应的患儿的合并症。

6. 排尿期膀胱尿道造影可用来诊断膀胱输尿管返流,以确定尿路感染的原因,但仅适用于有异常RBUS或复发性发热性UTI的儿童。

参考文献:

Urinary Tract Infection: Clinical Practice Guideline for the Diagnosis and Management of the Initial UTI in Febrile Infants and Children 2 to 24 Months. Subcommittee on Urinary Tract Infection, Steering Committee on Quality Improvement and Management. Pediatrics 2011; 595-610.

作者: Lauren Rice

儿科急诊

197. Pediatric Pneumonia

1. You have diagnosed an infant or child with pneumonia. How do you decide if they need admission?

2. The Pediatric Infectious Disease Society and the British Thoracic Society each have guidelines from 2011 to help with this decision.

3. The Pediatric Infectious Disease Society recommend inpatient therapy for the following

1) oxygen saturation <90%.

2) infants less than 3 – 6 months of age with bacterial infection being the likely etiology.

3) pneumonia from suspected or documented virulent pathogen such as CA-MRSA.

4) children in whom home care is questionable, outpatient follow-up is not available or who cannot comply with outpatient therapy.

4. The British Thoracic Society identify risk factors likely to require hospitalization:

1) oxygen saturation <92%.

2) respiratory rate >70 breaths/min (>50 breaths/min in older children).

3) significant tachycardia for level of fever.

4) prolonged capillary refill time >2 seconds.

5) breathing difficulty.

6) intermittent apnea.

7) not feeding or signs of dehydration.

8) chronic medical conditions/comorbidities.

Author: Mimi Lu

197. 小儿肺炎

1. 你刚刚诊断一个婴儿或儿童患有肺炎，如何决定患儿是否需要住院治疗？

2. 美国儿科感染病学会和英国胸科学会在2011年发表的指南将有助于你的决定。

3. 美国儿科感染病学会住院治疗标准

1）氧饱和度低于90%；

2）3~6个月婴儿高度怀疑有细菌感染；

3）由可疑或证实的恶性病原菌（如院外获得的MRSA）导致的肺炎；

4）不能落实可靠的家庭治疗，不能随诊，不能遵守门诊治疗方案。

4. 英国胸科学会明确了需要住院的几个危险因素

1）氧饱和度低于92%；

2）呼吸频率＞70次/分（大一点的小孩超过50次/分）；

3）与发病程度不相符的心动过速；

4）毛细血管充盈时间超过2秒钟；

5）呼吸困难；

6）间歇性呼吸停止；

7）不能进食或有脱水征；

8）有慢性疾病或合并症。

参考文献：

"The Management of Community-Acquired Pneumonia in Infants and Children Older Than 3 Months of Age：Clinical Practice Guidelines by the Pediatric Infectious Diseases Society and the Infectious Diseases Society of America"

"Guidelines for the management of community acquired pneumonia in children：update 2011" BTS

http：//www. brit-thoracic. org. uk/Portals/0/Guidelines/Pneumonia/CAP% 20children% 20October% 202011. pdf

作者：**Mimi Lu**

儿科急诊

198. Varicella-related stroke

1. Acute ischemic stroke occurs in 3.3/100, 000 children per year. Up to 30% of these are caused by varicella. This can be diagnosed if the patient has had varicella infection within the past 12 months, has a unilateral stenosis of a great vessel, and has a positive PCR or IgG from the CSF.

2. Treatment includes anticoagulation, acyclovir for at least 7 days and steroids for 3 – 5 days.

3. Outcome is normally good and spontaneous improvement can be seen.

4. Inflammation of other arteries, including other areas of the brain, can also be seen. Treatment options for this can include high dose glucocorticoids and possibly immunosuppresive agents.

Author: Jennifer Guyther

198. 与水痘有关的脑卒中

1. 每年 100 000 名儿童中会有 3.3 名患急性缺血性脑卒中，其中高达 30% 是由水痘引起的。如有下列情况可以确诊：患者在过去 12 个月内有过水痘感染史，单侧大血管狭窄，脑脊液中 PCR 或 IgG 阳性。

2. 治疗包括抗凝，至少 7 天的阿昔洛维和 3～5 天激素。

3. 患者预后良好，也常见自发性好转。

4. 其他动脉包括其他的大脑区域也可以发生炎症。治疗方案包括给予高剂量的糖皮质激素和免疫抑制药。

参考文献：

Simma et al. Therapy in pediatric stroke. Eur J Pediatr. Published online 06 November 2012.

作者：Jennifer Guyther

199. Pediatric ultrasound and appendicitis

1. An overweight 5 year old male presents with acute onset abdominal pain that localizes to the right lower quadrant. What are some causes of a limited or nondiagnostic ultrasound study in children?

2. Acute appendicitis is a time sensitive diagnosis. Ultrasound is frequently used as the initial diagnostic imaging in children. There are several reasons why the appendix may not be visualized, including retro-cecal location, normal appendix, perforation, and inflammation around the distal tip. An additional clinical predictor associated with poor or inconclusive ultrasound results in appendicitis is increased BMI (body mass index).

3. A study examining 263 pediatric patients found when BMI > 85th percentile and clinical probability of appendicitis was < 50%, 58% of ultrasounds were nondiagnostic. Children with a BMI < 85th percentile and clinical probability of appendicitis was < 50%, had nondiagonstic scans 42% of the time. These trends were also mimicked in the patients with a higher clinical probability of appendicitis. In the child with a nondiagnostic ultrasound, options include observation and repeat ultrasound scan or CT scan, both of which have associated risks.

Author: **Mimi Lu**

199. 儿科超声检查与阑尾炎

1. 一个体重超重的 5 岁男孩，因急性右下腹痛就诊。造成超声检查在儿童中受限或不能确诊的原因有哪些?

2. 急性阑尾炎需要快速诊断。超声在儿科患者中经常被用来作为初始诊断的影像检查手段。有几种原因可以来解释为什么有时候会看不到阑尾，包括盲肠后的位置、正常阑尾、穿孔和炎症发生在阑尾远端。另外一个造成超声检查结果质量不高或不能确定阑尾炎的临床预测指标是高 BMI(体重指数)。

3. 对 263 例小儿患者的一项研究发现，当 BMI >85 百分位且阑尾炎临床可能性 <50% 时，58% 的超声不能明确诊断。BMI <85 百分位而阑尾炎临床可能性 <50% 的儿童，有 42% 的超声检查不能明确诊断。在临床阑尾炎可能性很高的患者中也有类似趋势。对于超声不能明确诊断的孩子，可选择观察和重复超声波检查或 CT 扫描，当然这两者都有一定的风险。

参考文献：

Schuh S, et al. Predictors of non-diagnostic ultrasound scanning in children with suspected appendicitis. J Pediatr. 2011 Jan; 158(1): 112 – 8.

作者：Mimi Lu

儿科急诊

200. Acute Diarrhea

1. Diarrhea lasting less than 14 days.

2. In children, almost all diarrhea is due to an infectious agent.

3. Most etiologies are self-limited and do not need further evaluation except in the following conditions:

1) infants <2 months of age.

2) gross blood in stool.

3) WBC's on microscopic exam of stool.

4) toxic-appearance.

5) immunocompromised child.

6) diarrhea developing while an inpatient.

4. Therapy is aimed at oral rehydration and providing nutrional needs.

5. ORT is best with commerical formulations specific for this as most other clear liquids (juice, sodas) are hypertonic and have excess glucose resulting in ongoing diarrhea-like stools.

6. After rehydration, resume the child's normal diet.

Author: Rose Chasm

200. 急性腹泻

1. 腹泻持续时间少于 14 天。

2. 在儿童中, 几乎所有的腹泻都是由于感染性因素造成的。

3. 大多数病因是自愈性的, 但下列情况需要进一步的检查

1) < 2 月龄婴儿;

2) 肉眼血便;

3) 大便镜检有 WBC;

4) 有全身中毒表现;

5) 免疫功能低下的孩子;

6) 住院期间出现腹泻。

4. 治疗目的是口服补液和保证营养的需求。

5. 最好使用为这一目的设计的商品化的配方, 口服补液盐(ORT), 因为多数其他液体(果汁, 苏打水)都是高渗并含有较高的葡萄糖, 可能导致持续性与腹泻类似的大便。

6. 补液后, 患儿可恢复正常饮食。

参考文献:

MedStudy Pediatrics Board Review Core Curriculum

作者: **Rose Chasm**

急诊操作
Emergency Procedures

201. Lidocaine with Epinephrine and it use on Fingers and Toes

1. It has been taught for a long time that Lidocaine with Epinephrine should not be used on fingers, toes, ears and nose due to the risk of vasoconstricition/vasospasm and possible digitial infarcation.

2. The short story is that this practice is not supported by the literature, and there are now numerous publications that have shown that lidocaine with epinephrine is safe for use on the finger tips.

3. It turns out the original case reports were submitted with procaine and epinephrine and not lidocaine with epinephrine. Most of the cases of digital infarction where with straight procaine that is now thought to have been contaiminated or too acidic pH close to 1 when injected.

4. The effects of epinephrine last approximately 6 hours. This time is well within the accepted limit of ischemia for fingers that has been established in digitial replanation.

5. So why use Lidocaine with Epinephrine:

1) Provides a longer period of anesthesia.

2) Decreases bleeding which.

3) Improves visualization of tendons and underlying structures.

4) Makes repairs easier.

5) Decreases need for a tourniquet.

Author: Michael Bond

201. 含肾上腺素的利多卡因及其在指趾麻醉的应用

1. 长时间以来认为，含有肾上腺素的利多卡因不能用于手指、脚趾、耳朵和鼻子的麻醉，因为它可使血管收缩/痉挛，进而导致手指栓塞。

2. 这种临床习惯并没有文献支持，相反，最近有许多文献显示含肾上腺素的利多卡因在手指的麻醉中是安全的。

3. 原来最开始的病例报告都是用的含肾上腺素的普鲁卡因，而不是利多卡因。现在认为很多手指栓塞的病例是因为普鲁卡因被污染或酸性太强，注射后pH 接近 1。

4. 肾上腺素的作用大约持续 6 小时，断指再植证实，这个时间是在造成手指缺血的可允许范围内的。

5. 使用含肾上腺素的利多卡因原因：

1）提供较长的麻醉效果；

2）减少出血；

3）清楚地看到肌腱和周围结构；

4）容易修复；

5）减少对止血带的需求。

参考文献：

Thomson CJ, Lalonde DH, Denkler KA, Feicht AJ. A critical look at the evidence for and against elective epinephrine use in the finger. Plast Reconstr Surg. Jan 2007；119（1）：260 – 266.

作者：**Michael Bond**

急诊操作

202. Needle Decompression for Tension Pneumothorax (new site)

Needle Decompression—Are we Teaching the Right Location?

1. Tension pneumothorax frequently results in circulatory collapse and may lead to cardiopulmonary arrest.

2. In the event that tube thoracostomy cannot be immediately performed, traditional teaching is to perform needle decompression in the second intercostal space, mid-clavicular line using a 5 cm angiocath needle.

3. Recent literature, however, has challenged the traditional location for needle decompression. In fact, researchers found:

1) Needles placed in the second intercostal space often failed to enter the chest cavity and relieve tension physiology.

2) Needles placed in the fifth intercostal space in the anterior axillary line were more likely to enter the chest cavity with a lower failure rate.

4. Take Home Point: It may be time to reconsider the optimal position for needle decompression of tension pneumothorax.

Author: Michael Winters

202. 张力性气胸穿刺减压的新位置

穿刺减压——我们教的位置正确吗?

1. 张力性气胸常导致循环衰竭和心跳呼吸骤停。

2. 在不能立即放置胸导管的情况下,传统的穿插减压点是在第二肋间隙和锁骨中线交叉点插入一个5厘米的套管针。

3. 但是,近期文献对穿刺减压的传统位置提出了疑问。实际上,科研人员发现:

1) 在第二肋间隙放置穿刺针,经常不能进入胸腔从而解除高张的生理状态。

2) 在第五肋间隙和腋前线交叉点进针,更容易进入胸腔,失败率低。

4. 要点

可能是时候考虑张力性气胸穿刺减压的最佳位置了。

参考文献:

Inaba K, et al. Optimal positioning for emergent needle thoracostomy: A cadaver-based study. J Trauma 2011; 71: 1099 – 1103.

Inaba K, et al. Radiologic evaluation of alternative sites for needle decompression of tension pneumothorax. Arch Surg 2012; 147: 813 – 818.

Martin M, et al. Does needle decompression provide adequate and effective decompression of tension pneumothorax? J Trauma 2012; 73: 1412 – 1417.

作者: Michael Winters

急诊操作

203. Lumbar punctures and ultrasound?

1. Infant lumbar puncture is often difficult and may require repeated attempts. The traditional body positioning is lateral decubitus. Previous studies have examined the safety of having the patient in a sitting position, and neonatal studies have suggested that the subarachnoid space increases in size as the patient is moved to the seated position.

2. A study by Lo et al published looked to see if the same held true in infants.

3. 50 healthy infants less then 4 months old had the subarachnoid space measured by ultrasound between L3 – L4 in 3 positions: lateral decubitus, 45 degree tilt and sitting upright.

4. This study found that the size of the subarachnoid space did not differ significantly between the 3 positions.

5. Authors postulated that a reason for increase sitting LP success rate that had been reported in anestesia literature with tilt position could be due to other factors such as increased CSF pressure, intraspinous space widening or improved landmark identification.

Author: Jennifer Guyther

203.腰椎穿刺和超声

1. 婴儿腰椎穿刺往往是困难的，可能需要多次尝试。传统的体位是侧卧位。以往的研究已经检查了让患者坐着的安全性。有研究认为，新生儿在坐位状态下其蛛网膜下腔体积增大。

2. Lo 等人发表了一项研究，明确这一现象在婴儿中也是成立的。

3. 研究对象为 50 个健康的小于 4 个月的婴儿，对其 L3 – L4 之间的蛛网膜下腔的体积用超声在侧卧位、45 度倾斜位和正坐位分别进行了测量。

4. 研究发现，蛛网膜下腔的体积在 3 个位置之间没有显著不同。

5. 作者推测，麻醉杂志报告的坐位可增加腰穿成功率，可能是由于其他因素造成的，如脑脊液压力增高、脊突间间隙增宽或表面标记更明显。

参考文献：

Sitting or Tilt Position for Infant Lumbar Puncture Does Not Increase Ultrasound Measurements of Lumbar Subarachnoid Space Width. PediatrEmer Care 2013；29：588 – 591.

作者：**Jennifer Guyther**

急诊操作

204. Tranexamic Acid in Anterior Epistaxis

1. Tranexamic Acid (TXA) topically applied was compared to anterior nasal packing in 216 patients with acute anterior epistaxis. Cotton pledgets (15 cm) soaked in injectable TXA (500 mg/5 ml) were inserted into the bleeding nostril and removed after bleeding had arrested. This was compared to standard anterior packing.

2. RESULTS 结果:

	TXA	鼻前填塞
10 分钟内出血停止的比例(%)	71%	31.2%
2 小时后出院	95.3%	6.4%
24 小时后再出血	4.7%	11%
患者满意度(最高 10 分)	8.5	4.4

3. Bottom line:

topical tranexamic acid looks promising for control of uncomplicated anterior epistaxis.

Author: Ellen Lemkin

204. 氨甲环酸在鼻前出血中的应用

1. 在 216 例急性鼻前出血患者中，比较氨甲环酸(TXA)局部应用与鼻前填塞。将浸泡过注射用 TXA(500 mg/5 mL)棉拭子(15 厘米)插入出血的鼻孔，在出血停止后取出，将其与标准的鼻前填塞进行比较。

2. RESULTS 结果

	TXA	鼻前填塞
10 分钟内出血停止的比例(%)	71%	31.2%
2 小时后出院	95.3%	6.4%
24 小时后再出血	4.7%	11%
患者满意度(最高 10 分)	8.5	4.4

3. 要点

TXA 在控制单纯鼻前庭出血时是有效的。

参考文献：

Zahed R, Moharamzadeh P, AlizadeArasi S, Ghasemi A, Saeedi M. A new and rapid method for epistaxis treatment using injectable form of tranexamic acid topically: a randomized controlled trial. AJEM 2013 (31): 1389 - 1392.

作者: Ellen Lemkin

205. Lidocaine after IO Line Placement

1. Intraosseus (IO) access has become quite popular in critically ill patients requiring immediate resuscitation. In a patient responsive to pain, however, pain and discomfort is associated with the force of high-volume infusion through the established line.

1) Before flushing the line, consider administering preservative-free 2% lidocaine (without epinephrine) for patients responsive to pain prior to flush.

2) The suggested dose is 20 – 40 mg (1 – 2 mL) of the 2% lidocaine, followed by the 10 mL saline flush.

2. If preservative-free 2% lidocaine is not stocked in your ED, now is the time to consider adding it.

Author: Bryan Hayes

205.髓内通路放置后的利多卡因应用

1.在需要紧急复苏的危重患者的抢救中,骨髓内通道的应用已非常普遍。但是,对于一个对疼痛有感觉的患者,疼痛和不适可能会增加快速液体复苏的压力。

1)在冲洗髓内通道前,对有疼痛感的患者,可考虑注射无防腐剂的2%利多卡因(无肾上腺素)。

2)建议剂量是2%的利多卡因20~40 mg(1~2 mL),然后再用10 mL生理盐水冲管。

2.如果你们科里没有储存无防腐剂的2%的利多卡因,现在应该把它加上了。

参考文献:

Fowler RL, Pierce, Nazeer S, et al. Powered intraosseous insertion provides safe and effective vascular access for emergency patients. Ann Emerg Med 2008; 52(4): S152.

Ong MEH, Chan YH, Oh JJ, et al. An observational, prospective study comparing tibial and humeral intraosseus access using EZ-IO. Am J Emerg Med 2009; 27(1): 8 – 15. [PMID 19041528]

作者: Bryan Hayes

急诊操作

206. Hematoma Block

1. Provides good aesthesia for reduction of fractures. Onset in approximately 5 minutes

2. Benefits: No need for NPO, simple and easy to perform & can be done without additional personnel (unlike w/ procedural sedation)

3. Contraindications: Open fractures, dirty or infected overlying skin

1) Identify fracture site with x-ray and palpation.

2) Clean skin w/ Betadine.

3) Insert needle into the hematoma. Confirm placement by aspirating blood.

4) Inject anesthetic (lidocaine 1 or 2%) into the fracture cavity and adjacent periosteum.

Author: Brian Corwell

206. 血肿部位局麻

1. 可为骨折复位提供满意的麻醉效果，大概在 5 分钟内起效。
2. 优点：不需要禁食，操作简单容易，不需要有助手(与镇静操作不同)。
3. 禁忌证：开放性骨折，覆盖皮肤不干净或有感染。
1) 通过 X 线和触诊找到骨折部位；
2) 局部碘酒消毒；
3) 将针头刺入血肿，可通过回吸到血来证实位置的准确；
4) 将麻醉剂(1% ~2% 的利多卡因)注入到骨折间隙和骨膜。

参考文献：

http：//www. youtube. com/watch？ v = tjnsdjfwMmY

作者： **Brian Corwell**

207. Local anesthetics in pediatric patients

1. In children, it is important to consider the maximum doses of local anesthetics when performing a laceration repair or painful procedure like abscess drainage. If there are multiple lacerations, or large lacerations, it may be possible to exceed those doses if one is not careful.

Max doses of common anesthetics:

(1) Lidocaine WITHOUT epinephrine −4 mg/kg (0. 4 mL/kg of 1% lidocaine).

(2) Lidocaine WITH epinephrine −7 mg/kg (0. 7 mL/kg of 1% lidocaine).

(3) Bupivicaine WITHOUT epinephrine −2 mg/kg (0. 8 mL/kg of 0. 25% bupivicaine).

(4) Bupivicaine WITH epinephrine − 3 mg/kg (1. 2 mL/kg of 0. 25% bupivicaine).

2. Pearls

For added safety, some advocate not exceeding 80% of the max dose in children <8 years of age.

3. Higher concentration of lidocaine beyond 1% does not improve the time of onset or duration of action and may increases the risk of toxicity.

4. The addition of epinephrine increases the maximum dose and duration of action, but may be more painful during infiltration.

5. If the repair requires large amount of local anesthetic, consider doing an regional block.

Author: Mimi Lu

207.局部麻醉药在儿科中的应用

1.对于儿童来说，在做撕裂伤的修复或像脓肿引流这样易引发痛苦的操作时，一定要考虑到局部麻醉药的最大剂量。如有多发或大的撕裂伤，不小心很可能会超过剂量。

常用局部麻醉药的最大剂量

(1)无肾上腺素的利多卡因：4 mg/kg(0.4 mL/kg 的 1% 利多卡因)。

(2)有肾上腺素的利多卡因：7 mg/kg(0.7 mL/kg 的 1% 利多卡因)。

(3)无肾上腺素的布比卡因：2 mg/kg(0.8 mL/kg 的 0.25% 布比卡因)。

(4)有肾上腺素的布比卡因：3 mg/kg(1.2 mL/kg 的 0.25% 布比卡因)。

2.要点

为安全起见，建议对 8 岁以下的儿童不要超过 80% 的最大剂量。

3.浓度在 1% 以上的利多卡因并不能改善麻醉药起效或作用时间，反而有增加毒性的危险。

4.加入肾上腺素虽然可增加最大量和延长作用时间，但在注射时可能会更疼。

5.如修复需要大剂量的局部麻醉药，要考虑进行局部神经阻滞。

作者：Mimi Lu

灾难医学
Disaster Medicine

208. Pediatric Care in Disasters

1. General Information

1) 50% of victims in man-made and natural disasters are children.

2) In low and middle income countries (where 95% of disasters occur), children are particularly vulnerable.

2. Early responders must be well versed in caring for pediatric diarrheal disease, acute respiratory tract infections, measles, malaria, severe bacterial infections, malnutrition, micronutrient deficiencies, injuries, burns and poisonings with few resources.

3. Pediatric specific triage systems have been developed to aid in resource allocation during mass casualty responses.

4. Pediatric patients are singularly vulnerably to exploitation, abuse and trafficking during disaster, particularly when they are separated from their families.

5. Bottom Line:

Many US based emergency medicine physicians are keen to respond to international disasters. A clear understanding about the particular risks to children during disaster response are critical in order to care for the most vulnerable of disaster victims.

Author: Andrea Tenner

208. 灾难中的儿童救护

1. 一般资料

1）在人为和自然灾害中，50％的受害者是儿童。

2）在低到中等收入国家（95％的灾害发生地），儿童特别容易受到伤害。

早期救援者必须了解在资源不充足情况下，如何救治小儿腹泻、急性呼吸道感染、麻疹、疟疾、严重的细菌感染、营养不良、微量元素缺乏、受伤、烧伤和中毒。

3. 针对小儿的分流系统已经建立，以帮助在发生大规模人员伤亡时的资源分配。

4. 在灾难过程中，小儿患者最容易被利用、虐待和贩卖，尤其是当他们与家人失散后。

5. 要点

许多美国急诊医师都热衷于参加国际灾害救援。为了照顾最脆弱的灾民，救灾期间清楚地了解与儿童有关的特定风险是至关重要的。

参考文献：

Rothstein，D. Pediatric Care in Disasters. Pediatrics. 2013，132：25.

https：//umem. org/educational_pearls/2225/.

作者：Andrea Tenner

灾
难
医
学

209. Saving lives in a disaster

1. Background Information:

Ever wonder what you would do if you were the first on scene after the earthquake in Haiti or in the Superdome as Hurricaine Katrina survivors started to arrive? How could you save the most lives? As is typical of emergency medicine, blood and gore tend to get the most attention, but if you want to save lives you have to think about what is the greatest life threat. In a large-scale disaster, it turns out, lack of water and abundance of feces kill the most, the fastest and need to be addressed first.

2. The Sphere Project Handbook

1) one of the core documents of humanitarian response.

2) outlines what should be done to save the most lives in the first days, weeks, and months of a disaster.

3) available free online (see reference below).

3. Pertinent Conclusions: (need-to-know recommendations for the first few days)

1) Water: 15L/person/day (any quality—sanitize as per our previous pearl).

2) Latrines: max 20 people/latrine, < 50 m from dwellings, > 30 m from water sources.

What kind?

(1) First 2 – 3 days: demarcated defecation area.

(2) days – 2 months: trench latrines (shallow trenches to defecate in).

4. Other hygiene

1) Solid waste disposal: one 100L refuse container/10 households, emptied at least 2x/week.

2) Dead bodies: dispose of according to local custom. Generally not an immediate source of infection.

3) Shelter: > 3.5 sq. meters/person of covered floor space.

5. Bottom Line

People's need for water and defecation will not stop in a disaster and too little water and too much excrement are the greatest immediate life threats to disaster survivors. Plan to deal with these early to save the most lives.

Author: Andrea Tenner

209. 在灾难时如何拯救最多的生命？

1. 背景资料

你想过没有，如果你在海地地震或卡特里娜飓风后第一个到达现场，你会做什么？你如何才能抢救最多的生命？与急诊医学的典型例子一样，出血最容易引人注意，但是你如果要抢救生命，你必须要考虑什么是最威胁生命的？在发生大规模灾难时，实际上缺水和大量的粪便将在第一时间内夺去最多的生命，必须在第一时间解决。

2. 全球计划手册

1）人类救援反应的关键文件之一。

2）描述了在灾害的第一天、第一周和第一月内如何拯救最多的生命。

3）可在网上免费查到（见下面的参考文献）。

3. 有关的结论（前几天内需要知道的建议）

1）水：每人每天 15 升（任何质量的水饮用前须按前面的要求进行消毒处理）。

2）厕所：最多每 20 个人一个厕所，离住处 50 米内，离水源 30 米外。

具体是什么样的？

（1）在头 2~3 天：划定排粪区域。

（2）几天~2 月：挖出厕所（排便的浅沟）。

4. 其他卫生方面

1）固体废物处理. 每 10 家要有一个 100 升的废物桶，每周至少清理 2 次。

2）尸体。根据当地习俗处理，一般来说不是立即感染的原因。

3）庇护所。平均每人要有至少 3.5 平方米地面面积。

5. 要点

人对水和排便的需求并没有因为灾难的发生而停止，对幸存者来说，缺水和大量的排泄物是最致命的因素。

参考文献：

The Sphere Project. Sphere Handbook: Humanitarian Charter and Minimum Standards in Disaster Response, 2011, 2011, ISBN 92 – 9139 – 097 – 6, available at: http://www.sphereproject.org/handbook/

作者：**Andrea Tenner**

灾难医学

493

210. What injuries do you see after an explosion?

Clinical Pearl: What injuries do you see after an explosion?

1. Explosions can cause a complex series of injuries, which may includesubtle or delayed findings. Repeated evaluations, such as serialabdominal exams, may be required.

2. Blast injuries are divided into 4 categories:

1) Primary blast injuries: Injury from blast wave over-pressure. Found in gasfilled structures (ear, lung, hollow organs).

2) Secondary blast injuries: Injury from thrown objects (primarilypenetrating trauma, but may blunt).

3) Tertiary blast injuries: Injuries from patient being thrown by blast wave (blunt trauma).

4) Miscellaneous (quaternary) blast injuries: Injuries from other causes, such as burns, crush injuries, rhabdomyolysis, and toxic chemicals.

3. The most common primary blast injury is tympanic membrane rupture.

Author: Jon Mark Hirshon

美
国
急
诊
临
床
必
知
200
招

210. 爆炸事故会造成什么样的损伤？

爆炸事故会造成什么样的损伤？

1.爆炸事故会造成一系列的复合伤，包括潜在的或迟发的。需要进行包括系统腹部检查在内的重复性评估。

2.冲击伤分为四类：

1)原发性冲击伤。由冲击波直接对含有气体的器官造成的损伤，如耳、肺和空腔脏器。

2)二级冲击伤。由飞来的物体造成的外伤(主要是穿透伤，也可造成钝挫伤)。

3)三级冲击伤。由于患者被气流掀翻后造成的外伤。

4)其他(四级)冲击伤。由其他原因所造成的外伤，如烧伤、挤压伤、横纹肌溶解症和毒性化学物质。

3.最常见的原发性冲击伤是鼓膜破裂。

参考文献：

http：//emergency.cdc.gov/masscasualties/blastessentials.asp

作者：**Jon Mark Hirshon**

其他

Miscellaneous

211. Radiation Risk?

1. Risk is based on acute exposure and is extrapolated largely from atomic bomb survivors.

2. Effective radiation dose = Sievert (Sv)

3. Adults

1) Lifetime Attributable Risk of Cancer 1 : 1000 at 10 mSv.

2) Lifetime Attributable Risk of Cancer Mortality 1 : 2000 at 10 mSv.

3) Risk is Cumulative.

4. Pediatrics

1) Lifetime Attributable Risk of Cancer is greater than for adults and is age-dependent.

2) Lifetime Attributable Risk of Cancer Mortality 1 : 1000 at 10 mSv.

5. Common Effective Dose Estimates (mSv)

6. Note that it doesn't take very much radiation to reach the 10 mSv level!

7. Bottom line: CT if you need to, but carefully consider whether it is worth it or not

Background radiation 宇宙辐射	3.5/year 3.5/年
CXR 胸片	0.1
Head, Face CT 头, 面 CT	2
Neck, Cervical Spine CT 颈部, 颈椎 CT	2
Chest, Thoracic Spine CT 胸部, 胸椎 CT	8
Abdomen CT 腹部 CT	7.5
Pelvis CT 盆腔 CT	7.5
Abdomen/Pelvis, Lumbar Spine CT 腹/盆, 腰椎 CT	15
Extremity CT 肢体 CT	0.5

Author: Rob Rogers

211. 放射性检查的危害

1. 放射性检查的危害主要是基于短时间内暴露于辐射环境，大部分的结论来源于原子弹爆炸的幸存者。

2. 有效放射量的单位希沃特(Sv)。

3. 成人

1) 10 mSv 可致癌症发病率增加 1/1000；

2) 10 mSv 可致癌症死亡率增加 1/2000。

3) 危险程度具有累加效应。

4. 儿童

1) 导致一生中癌症的发病率要比成人高，并与年龄相关；

2) 10 mSv 可致癌症死亡率增加 1/1000；

5. 常见有效剂量的估计值(mSv)

Background radiation 宇宙辐射	3.5/year 3.5/年
CXR 胸片	0.1
Head, Face CT 头，面 CT	2
Neck, Cervical Spine CT 颈部，颈椎 CT	2
Chest, Thoracic Spine CT 胸部，胸椎 CT	8
Abdomen CT 腹部 CT	7.5
Pelvis CT 盆腔 CT	7.5
Abdomen/Pelvis, Lumbar Spine CT 腹/盆，腰椎 CT	15
Extremity CT 肢体 CT	0.5

6. 请注意，并不需要接受太多的射线就可达到 10 mSv 的水平！

7. 要点

如有必要可做 CT，但请仔细考虑是否值得。

作者：**Rob Rogers**

其他

212. Medscape's 2013 Emergency Physician Lifestyle Report?

1. Medscape's 2013 Physician Lifestyle Report provides physicians with insight from 24, 000 US physicians across 24 medical specialties on how burnout may affect their lifestyle choices and experiences. Burnout was defined as having one of the following symptoms: loss of enthusiasm for work, feelings of cynicism, and a low sense of personal accomplishment.

2. EM specialists suffered the most burnout among physicians (51%), followed closely by critical care physicians (50%). Others at the top of the list are family physicians, internists, and general surgeons. Surprisingly, pediatricians were among the least burned-out specialists, along with rheumatologists, psychiatrists, and pathologists.

3. EM physicians ranked 12th in the severity of burnout, with a mean severity score of 3.8, with 1 being burnout that does not interfere with their lives and 7 being so severe that they are thinking of leaving medicine.

4. The 2 top-rated stressors were "too many bureaucratic tasks" and "too many difficult patients. " The least important stressors for EM physicians were "difficult employer," "difficult colleagues or staff," and "income not high enough. "

5. A slightly higher percentage (52%) of male EM docs reported burnout.

6. Mid-career EM physicians experienced the most burnout.

7. EM physicians who said they felt burned out at work were more likely to feel burned out outside of work.

8. About 43% of burned-out emergency doctors take less than 2 week vacation each year compared with 25% of their happier peers.

9. Burnout EM physicians were less likely to volunteer, exercise, and have adequate savings.

Author: Feng Xiao

212. Medscape 2013 年急诊医生生活方式报告

1. Medscape 2013 年医师生活方式报告提供了来自 24 个医学专科的 24,000 名美国医师对职业倦怠如何影响他们的生活方式的选择和经验。职业倦怠定义为具有下列症状之一：丧失对工作的热情、愤世嫉俗和没有个人成就感。

2. 急诊科医生在所有医生中是最容易患职业倦怠的(51%)，紧随其后的是重症医学科医生(50%)。其他名列前茅的是家庭医生、内科医生和普通外科医生。令人惊讶的是，与风湿科、精神科和病理科医生一样，儿科医生是非常不容易出现职业倦怠的。

3. 急诊科医生职业倦怠的严重程度排在第 12 位，平均严重度评分为 3.8 分。评分标准为：1 分是虽有职业倦怠但不干扰他们的生活；7 分是职业倦怠非常严重以至于他们正在考虑离开医疗岗位。

4. 影响急诊医生职业倦怠最大的压力有"太多的官僚作风"和"有麻烦的患者太多"。对急诊医生来说最不重要的压力源是"讨厌的雇主"，"麻烦的同事或工作人员"和"收入不够高"。

5. 男性急诊医生表现职业倦怠的比例稍高(52%)。

6. 中期职业生涯中的急诊医生最常最容易出现职业倦怠。

7. 有职业倦怠感的急诊医生通常也更容易在工作以外表现出倦怠情绪。

8. 与他们快乐的同行相比(25%)，大约 43% 的有职业倦怠感的急诊医生每年休假不到 2 周。

9. 职业倦怠的急诊医生不太可能做义工、锻炼身体和有足够的储蓄。

参考文献：

http://www.medscape.com/features/slideshow/lifestyle/2013/emergency-medicine

作者：Feng Xiao（肖锋）

其他

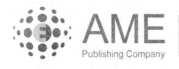

Academic Made Easy, Excellent and Enthusiastic

欲穷千里目，快乐搞学术